60 Years Living with Diabetes

In Spite of the Medical Profession

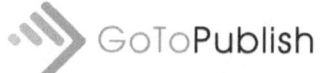

James Zajac

60 Years Living with Diabetes

In Spite of the Medical Profession

60 Years Living with Diabetes
Copyright © 2020 by James Zajac

Library of Congress Control Number: 2020905123
ISBN-13:   Paperback: 978-1-64749-011-9
           ePub: 978-1-64749-134-5

All rights reserved. No part of this publication may be reproduced, distributed, or transmitted in any form or by any means, including photocopying, recording, or other electronic or mechanical methods, without the prior written permission of the publisher or author, except in the case of brief quotations embodied in critical reviews and certain other noncommercial uses permitted by copyright law.

Although every precaution has been taken to verify the accuracy of the information contained herein, the author and publisher assume no responsibility for any errors or omissions. No liability is assumed for damages that may result from the use of information contained within.

Printed in the United States of America

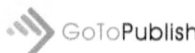

GoToPublish LLC
1-888-337-1724
www.gotopublish.com
info@gotopublish.com

Contents

Dedication vii
Introduction ix
Chapter One 1
Chapter Two 9
Chapter Three 18
Chapter Four 23
Chapter Five 44
Conclusion 76

Dedication

I dedicate this book to J. Deaver Alexander, MD, who was the only doctor in my sixty years with diabetes who understood anything about the disease and got me on the right track with managing my diabetes. If I had never had him for a doctor, I doubt I would still be alive to write this book, and I'm still going strong because of what I learned from him.

Introduction

I am seventy-three years old and became a diabetic when I was thirteen years old. My diabetes has been little more than a slight inconvenience during my sixty years with the disease in spite of the medical profession. I take between thirty and forty units of insulin a day, which consists of Humulin N and Humulin R. I was for a time taking Humalog and Lantus insulin. These two insulin, along with NovoLog, Apidra, and Levimir, are what I consider engineered insulin—insulin that are not natural but are designed by the pharmaceutical industry, which I believe have a detrimental effect in the treatment of diabetes, even though they make it easier to control your glucose levels. I will explain this in more depth toward the end of my history as a diabetic. Also as a diabetic, I take no drugs. Absolutely no drugs—none for blood pressure and no statin drugs. My cholesterol is usually around 180–190, and my blood pressure is 135 over 75, sometimes as high as 140. These readings are fine with me. They may not be with the doctors, but I'm in charge of my life, not them. Cholesterol at 180–190 is normal and has no need of being lower. There is certainly no need for it to be lower because I am a diabetic, in my opinion, and I sure don't need to be taking statin drugs. As far as my blood pressure goes, it's at the high limit. Ideally, I wish it was where it used to be when I was a young man (120 over 80), but I guess at seventy-three I should expect it to elevate. Although my blood pressure is at 130 to 140, and sometime it rises as high as 150 on rare occasions, I take care of it naturally. My energy level has already waned, and I don't need a lower amount of energy, which is what blood pressure medicine does to you. Besides, it used to be normal for older people's blood pressure to be 130 to 140, but the pharmaceutical industry decided that too much money was slipping through their fingers by letting that thinking persist. So they decided to scare everyone into thinking any blood pressure over 120 is high and dangerously so. It's bullshit. Blood pressure medicine causes more harm than 130 to 140 blood pressure will. Of course, 120 is ideal, but achieve it naturally and not through the pharmaceuticals. I take VitaOlive sold by Gold Leaf Nutritionals, but there are many other supplements out there for you to try. I take one capsule a day of the VitaOlive, although lately I have been thinking about taking the recommended two capsules a day because my blood pressure has climbed back up to 130–140.

Three things that I cherish immensely are freedom! Freedom! Freedom! For a while, when I was using the engineered insulin, I had lost some of my freedom to the doctors and insurance company. Humulin N and R insulin can be bought over the counter without a prescription, so I don't need the doctor anymore, and because I buy my insulin for twenty-five dollars a bottle, which is only five dollars over what my co-pay used to be, I don't need to be bothered with insurance. I buy all my diabetes supplies through my local Walmart pharmacy, including my insulin and also my glucose monitoring supplies. At Walmart, my glucose test strips cost me seventeen dollars for a hundred test strips. Last I checked, your typical pharmacy charges a little over a hundred dollars for the same amount of test strips, fifty-one dollars for Humulin N and R insulin, and one hundred twenty dollars for any of the engineered insulin, and most of them are a lot more and some of them have class-action lawsuits against them.

Concerning test strips, with my insurance company, my co-pay was twenty or thirty-five dollars if I used them up within a month. If I checked my glucose a bit more often than three times a day, I would be punished by the insurance company and have to co-pay thirty-five dollars. Through Walmart I pay seventeen dollars and I can monitor my glucose as often as I want without worrying about insurance. I consider Walmart a true friend to diabetics. I would also like to add that my co-pay for the engineered insulin was thirty-five dollars. So you see, I now don't need to bother with insurance or doctors for my diabetic supplies anymore. I have complete control over my diabetes as I see fit and am answerable to no one. Freedom!

Now you're probably wondering how I know that the quality or accuracy is not inferior to the more expensive brands. When I first started buying from Walmart, I checked the accuracy by comparing the readings to what I used to use, which was OneTouch Ultra. My readings were very close, and I felt Walmart's were more consistent. I would do three readings, one right after another, and have a variation of three or four points. I performed this analysis with my glucose somewhere around one hundred. Comparisons with OneTouch Ultra were also done with my glucose near two hundred and were acceptable to me. I also used to compare a test strip from an old container with a strip from a new container to see how much they varied. It was around three points. Try that with any of your test strips that cost one dollar apiece. What I buy from Walmart is the ReliOn Confirm Micro brand. They work similarly to the FreeStyle Lite brand that is advertised on television. I test on my fingers; all I need is a small drop of blood, and I touch the test strip to it and it draws the blood right in. When I buy my insulin, I also buy Walmart's ReliOn brand, which is produced by Lilly. There are only three companies that produce insulin; Lilly is one of them and probably the largest. Walmart, I guess, deals directly with Lilly and can sell much cheaper. They have also received their insulin from Novo Nordisk.

If you haven't done the math yet on how much my diabetes costs me, let me add it up for you. I take R and N insulin, and a bottle of each type lasts me approximately two months. That comes to twelve bottles of insulin a year at twenty-five dollars a bottle—a total of $300 a year. My test strips cost me seventeen dollars for a box of one hundred. A box of one hundred lasts me almost a month, but not quite. I buy thirteen boxes a year at seventeen dollars, which comes to $221 a year. Usually I only need to check my glucose two or three times a day, but when I work out or exercise, I need to know where my glucose is before I start. I want it to be about 150 or higher so I don't crash during my workout or bike ride or swimming. So far my diabetes costs me $521 out of my own pocket. This amount is basically the same as if I used insurance to purchase everything.

My next expense is for the doctor and lab tests. I see my doctor at best once a year and sometimes every eighteen months. My doctor visit cost is seventy-five dollars, and the lab work requested used to cost the insurance company $466.25, but now I think it's over $1,000. All totaled, my diabetes costs me and my insurance company $1,521 per year. Now, out of the seventy-five dollars for the doctor visit, I have to co-pay twenty dollars. So that raises my yearly expenses to $541 and the insurance expenditures to $1,586. One other expense that I have is for insulin syringes. I use the disposable kind over and over, so a box of a hundred lasts me over a year and costs twenty dollars a box. That brings my total to $561 a year. Not bad for a seventy-two-year-old man who has lived with diabetes for sixty years and without the control of doctors. I would also like to add that I have all my toes, my kidneys function quite well, and my eyesight needs very little correction. I use to wear contacts, but I've had cataract surgery two years ago, and now I don't need any eyesight correction but reading glasses.

Right now I bet many of you are wondering why I worry about what I cost the insurance company. It's because I accept responsibility for everything that I do. The money that I cost the insurance company comes out of my pocket and that of everyone else who subscribes to the same insurance company, whether it is paid by your employer or by you.

Most everyone wants to be entitled to insurance coverage or have their medical bills covered by the government. Few people pay their medical costs themselves, and they also feel that as long as they don't have to pay anything except a co-pay, why worry about the expense? But it does come out of your pocket in elevated insurance premiums or, if you're on Medicaid or Medicare, out of higher taxes for those who pay taxes. I handle my medical well-being with great responsibility. I want proper and adequate care but at the lowest price possible, whether it is out of my pocket or the insurance company's pocket. Responsibility is something that few people, in today's world, concern themselves with, especially our politicians. That is why we are in such an economic mess today, and of course we have the liberal left who says, "Don't accept responsibility. The government will take care of you [and control your life]."

I have a book that I refer to occasionally called *Beat Diabetes Naturally*. In this book they give a statistic on how much diabetes costs this nation, which is $100 billion annually. They go on to say the average annual health-care cost of a diabetic is approximately $12,000, while health-care costs for a nondiabetic total about $3,000. My diabetes costs are less than half of the costs for the average adult without diabetes. This is something that I am very proud of, and I am even more proud of the fact that I have done it without the assistance of the medical profession.

Next, you're probably wondering how I can keep my diabetes in control or even know if it is under control when I see a doctor once a year at best. The only reason I see a doctor at all is for a yearly examination and to have the typical diabetes tests done so I can make sure I'm doing as well as I believe I am, and I don't leave it up to the doctor to make that determination. I always get my test results sent directly to me, and I review them myself and make my own determinations. I've had doctors overlook results because they lack concern with it or because they too briefly looked at the results in the first place. I can't emphasize enough the importance of getting your own copy of your test results. In the state of Pennsylvania, I spent ten years trying to get legislation passed so that I and everyone else don't have to ask a doctor's permission to see our own test results or get a copy of them. I had been denied my test results in the past and even had one doctor tell me that there were state and federal laws that prevented him from giving me any of my medical records. It took a long time, but somewhere around the turn of the century, the legislation was passed, and now the labs have to inform you that you are entitled to a copy of your test results to be sent directly to you.

Whenever I tell anyone about getting their test results sent to them directly, they almost always say their doctor will give them a copy if they ask for it. My response to them is always the same: "What's wrong with getting the results before you talk with your doctor? Then you know what questions you should be asking." This allows you to take control of your life rather than leaving it in control of the doctors. A doctor should be nothing more than an advisor and should not have complete control over your medical well-being. That control belongs in your hands and no one else's.

Back to why I see a doctor once a year at best. First off, I don't allow doctors to be involved with the control of my diabetes. That control is in my hands and my hands only. I decide how much insulin I will take each day, and I decide when it needs to be varied and by how much. I monitor my blood glucose and never ignore it, and it rarely reaches 200 or higher. A normal person's glucose is maintained between 70 and 110. I feel the closer you maintain your glucose to what is normal, the healthier you will stay, and allowing glucose levels to rise to the point that your kidneys are trying in vain to remove the excess glucose by dumping it into your urine is highly detrimental. It puts extra stress on your kidneys and affects your eyes. Excess glucose affects every part of your body where small capillaries are present. The smaller the capillaries, the more vulnerable to excess glucose. Sometimes after a meal, I check my urine for glucose to make sure my glucose is not rising up around 200. It's a very inexpensive test and not time-specific. It just lets me know if my glucose has risen up where I don't want it. For myself, I try to maintain my glucose between 70 and 150. The 150 is because your glucose is going to rise after meals, and that is usually how high mine rises. Because I know where my glucose levels are most of the time, I find it very unnecessary to spend any more time than once a year with a doctor. They never have any good advice or have done anything for me but take money from my pocket and put it in theirs.

Although I try to maintain my glucose as close to normal as possible and recommend it to all diabetics, you have to exercise caution in doing so because if you slip up and your glucose falls too low, you have the problem of hypoglycemic shock. Your glucose has fallen so low that your body is having problems functioning, especially the brain. So is the rest of your body, but in this situation, your brain is most important. Most importantly, you have to get in tune with your body. There are many little idiosyncrasies that will tell you when your glucose is getting low, and you have to pay attention to them and react to them. When my eyesight and my mind start playing tricks on me, I know my glucose is in the danger zone, but usually I can tell when it's low just by the way I feel. This is something that I can't describe. It is just something that you get to know. If you're ever tired and it's not normal, check your glucose. In the afternoon I sometimes unknowingly get tired and drift off to sleep because my glucose is low. Luckily my dog will wake me, and I correct the situation. These are some examples of how I pay attention to the control of my diabetes.

My diabetes is my diabetes! It's not a doctor's case of diabetes; it's my diabetes. It's up to me to control, and I don't let doctors interfere whatsoever. Everyone familiar with diabetes knows what an HGB A1c test is—or should. It determines how good your control of your glucose levels has been. The test measures how much glucose or blood sugar you have stuck to your red blood cells. Your red blood cells last an average of 90 to 120 days. Actually, it's the red pigment part of the cell that gets glycosylated with blood sugar and shows the average amount of blood sugar for the past three months. The last two times I have had my A1c checked, it was 6.1 both times, and going as far back as March of 2015, it was 5.8. Now I know there will be a lot of people, doctors especially, saying that I'm not being tested enough. As I have previously said, I have myself checked and tested once a year just to confirm that I'm doing as well as I believe I am. At 6.1, I would say I'm doing quite well, and to be tested any more often would be a great waste of my time and money.

The most important advice that I feel I have to offer, especially to young people who have become diabetics and even older people who have been diabetic for some time, is to accept that it is your diabetes and not the doctor's. The doctor should be an advisor to you and not be out to control you. A doctor should not be telling you to take a certain amount of insulin and to never deviate from it. That is the biggest and worst bunch of crap any doctor can tell you.

Diabetes is forever fluctuating, and no matter what the medical profession or anyone else says, it always will. There are just too many things that cause it to fluctuate: stress, a slight cold and especially a severe one, change in activity, fear, anxiety, anger, not only how much you eat but what you eat, and also what time of the month it is. Every diabetic I have talked to says that two weeks out of the month, it seems they can't do anything wrong, and the next two weeks they have a hard time doing anything right. With all these things affecting your control, how can any responsible doctor try to regiment your insulin dosages and your life in general? If this is the kind of doctor you presently have, dump him and find another one. When you go to the first appointment, don't give your insurance information or any money.

You will only have to spend a few minutes with the doctor to find out whether he is a good fit for you. If he is, then pay him or give him your insurance card. If he isn't, let him know you won't be wanting him for your doctor and get up and leave. All it has cost you is some time but no money. Don't let the doctors have their way with you. If they have their way, the only one who benefits from it is them and not you.

One more important piece of advice is to read as much as you can about diabetes. Buy books about diabetes, especially the ones about natural treatments of the disease. There are some very good books out about the treatment of diabetes naturally, such as *Diabetes without Drugs* by Suzy Cohen and *Beat Diabetes Naturally* by Michael Murray and Michael Lyon, although the latter may not be easily available because it was published in 2006. Both of these books recommend nutritional supplements and a nutritional approach to managing the disease. Although these two books are very good, the best book of all that I have come across is *The 30-Day Diabetes Cure* by Dr. Stefan Ripich, ND, CNP, and Jim Healthy. This book is a must-read for anyone with diabetes. It involves changing your eating habits and lifestyle to cure yourself of diabetes, and believe me, it is worth reading. If you don't know anything about nutritional supplements, all I have to say is that I believe in them emphatically and that it isn't going to hurt to at least familiarize yourself a little bit with nutritional supplements. The recommendation for supplements is starting to become more widespread among doctors but is still somewhat rare. After all, the American Medical Association (AMA) still has bogus reports printed in the newspapers about the benefits of nutritional supplements, calling them a waste of money. I have no kind words to say about the AMA and will have more to say about them in my conclusion at the end of the book.

A brief story on how I got involved with nutritional supplements: In my early years, all the way to my late twenties, I never took nutritional supplements. Poison ivy was always a problem for me, until one spring I decided to take a multivitamin pill that also had some minerals in it. That year my bouts with poison ivy were greatly diminished and haven't been a problem since, although I still get minor rashes. About fifteen years ago, I started taking a mineral supplement and am presently taking Ionic Mineral Complete by Pharm Origins, and now I don't get poison ivy at all—even after pulling it up with my hands. Of course I make sure I wash my hands afterward, but sometimes it is more than an hour afterward. The benefits from the minerals involved more than the poison ivy.

Any supplements that I take I have taken on my own without the advice or consent of doctors. My advice on nutritional supplements is if you have a problem and you think a particular supplement will do you some good, then try it. If you receive no benefit, stop taking it. It's rare that you will experience any side effects from them, and usually they're minor and insignificant effects such as soft stool or upset stomach, which is remedied by a reduction in the amount—or you can just stop taking it, and no harm done. There are plenty of natural healing remedies. There are books written by doctors on this subject, and the greatest advantage to them is that there are no bad side effects. With everything that the pharmaceutical industry produces, there are bad side effects, and many are life-threatening. So you can take the time and a small amount of money and buy a book written by an enlightened doctor and find a natural cure, or go to a regular doctor and get a prescription. Of course, you'll be rolling the dice—how lucky do you feel? If you go with the prescription, at least get the sheet that accompanies the prescription that they're supposed to give you and read about the side effects and all the different things you aren't supposed to be eating and things you're not supposed to do. Although I shove all doctors' advice aside and don't even consult with them, it's because I have never let them put me on any of their drugs, so I don't have to worry about reactions. If you are on other medications, it is advisable (and with some drugs, very important) that you consult with your doctor before trying anything. If you do consult with your doctor concerning another problem that you're having, don't let him give you another drug without first trying to resolve the problem naturally.

In ending my introduction, I would like to emphasize a few things. Don't just go to a doctor and let them have their way with you. Especially stay away from doctors who don't want to give you any freedom with your diabetes. There are doctors who believe that you have to learn to manage the disease yourself and that they can only offer advice and some direction on how to do it. I don't know how many of these doctors there are; I hope they are getting more plentiful, because that is the kind of doctor you want. Walk away from the rest. In the past I have always said you'll have to go through at least twenty doctors before you find a good one. You first have to have a doctor who will talk to you. If you have a doctor with whom you can't have a conversation, he is worthless. All he is going to do is give you orders and have control. You're the one who has to have control, not him. The best doctor I ever had was a doctor who had conversations with me about some things that weren't even pertinent to diabetes. He is the doctor to whom I have dedicated this book. I also had one other doctor whom I liked. He was an orthopedic doctor who treated a broken foot I had. He talked to me and joked with me without trying to control me. Too many want their patients to be like dogs in a lab experiment: be obedient, keep your mouth shut, and let them have their way with you.

I enjoy life; I work hard and I play hard. During the summer, I let my glucose drop so I can enjoy a dish of ice cream. I let it drop by taking the same amount of insulin as I normally take when I should take less because I'm going to be active that day. My glucose drops, and I make up for it by enjoying a dish of ice cream. It's not diabetic ice cream; it's regular ice cream. I also enjoy some ring bologna and cheese with a glass of wine in the evening, three or four times a week, and it doesn't send my glucose soaring. It stays just about the same for hours afterward. I avoid many of the highs and lows of diabetes by avoiding simple carbohydrates. When I make a sandwich, the bread I use is whole grain bread and not white bread. The more complex my carbohydrates are, the more stable my diabetes remains. I enjoy life like a normal person without diabetes does. I also consider the world a big playground, and if you're not having fun in it, it's because you're either lazy or stupid— usually it's a whole lot of both. So get outside and enjoy life. Diabetes should not be preventing you from it. Next is my history with diabetes, which should explain why I have so much contempt for the medical profession, especially the doctors.

A few last things I would like to say about nutritional supplements. Two that I don't believe further life for me would be possible without them and that I believe everyone should be taking. First is glycine, which is an amino acid that protects your kidneys. I take it because one day I was reading some information from the Joslin Clinic in Boston MA. They said they used glycine to benefit them in treating diabetics with kidney failure. So I thought if it is beneficial in the treatment of kidney failure why wouldn't it be beneficial in preventing kidney failure. I don't know when I started taking it, but I imagine it was at least ten years ago. It can be found in nutritional supplement stores, but not all of them carry it. Second is acetyl-L-carnitine with alpha-lipoic acid, which I buy at GNC stores. Carnitine is supposed to benefit your heart, and I was having chest pains—not severe ones but nevertheless annoying. I felt the annoying pains were caused by my heart and felt carnitine would correct the problem, which it did. The longer I took it the better things got. It took me over a year to completely get rid of the annoying pains, but now I'm completely free of them and would not live without either of these supplements.

Chapter One

The Beginning of My Diabetes

It was late fall of 1958, and I was twelve years old. I was a child whose knees had swelled up to the size of softballs. They were not painful, just uncomfortable. I showed my mother my knees, which alarmed her, so she took me to our family doctor. After he examined me, he asked if I had recently had a sore throat. I replied no, I hadn't, which was the truth. The doctor then talked to my mother and told her my knees were swollen because I had rheumatic fever, and it had given me a heart murmur also. He next convinced my mother that I had to have had strep throat because strep infections always precede rheumatic fever. My mother then became convinced by the doctor and tried to convince me that oh, yes, I had had strep throat, to which again I responded that no, I hadn't. I was not listened to because doctors never listen to their patients; they just paint their own scenario. In my case my mother agreed with him because after all, he was a doctor, and back then my mother, like many people, was in awe of doctors.

I was next sent home and had to stay in bed and was prescribed penicillin. The penicillin was taken orally, and the doctor said it was to prevent a recurrence of the sore throat that I never had. In defense of the doctor, penicillin was, and I believe still is, routinely prescribed for rheumatic fever patients because the medical profession says every case of rheumatic fever is preceded by a strep infection, some so slight that they weren't noticed. Of course we have to convince everyone that they need penicillin whether they do or not. The penicillin is only prescribed to prevent a recurrence of strep infection. This I didn't agree with, even as a twelve-year-old. For about the next three months, I had to stay in bed and wasn't allowed to sit up except to eat. I was allowed to get up with assistance to go to the toilet to defecate, but I had to urinate in a bottle. I don't recall how quickly the swelling in my knees went down. It seems to me it took probably a month, but the heart murmur took more time. Around the end of February, my doctor made one of his calls to see how I was doing. He said I was doing well and that I could start getting up but had to keep it to a light amount. Because I had to urinate in a bottle while flat on my back, one had been left on the floor next to my bed. My mother picked it up to empty it while the doctor was still there and noticed my urine was cloudy, so she showed it to the doctor. He checked my urine and found that the cloudiness was from glucose in my urine and that now I was a diabetic. This was shortly after my thirteenth birthday. The number seven is considered a lucky number and thirteen an unlucky number—well, it sure was unlucky for me.

Now I was a diabetic. I was immediately put on about twenty units of insulin. The insulin was called Iletin. It is no longer produced today. I was also required to test my urine at least four times a day.

The next irritation was caused by the AMA and their recommended treatment of diabetes. Testing how much sugar was being spilled in my urine had to be done with Benedict's solution because it had to be lab-accurate results, and only Benedict's solution was acceptable for testing. At this point, I would also like to point out that before 1980, the only way to monitor your diabetes was by testing your urine to see how much glucose was being removed from your blood by your kidneys and dumped in your urine. Blood glucose monitoring wasn't made available to diabetics until around 1980.

Testing with Benedict's solution meant using a test tube and filling it with a specific amount of Benedict's and a certain amount of urine. Next I had to put a kettle of water on the stove, bring it to a boil, and place the test tube in the boiling water for five minutes. During the five minutes, the Benedict's and urine solution would change color, and at the end of the five minutes, the test tube was to be removed and the color checked to determine the amount of sugar in my urine. I was allowed to collect my urine samples and test them separately, but three or four at a time. Benedict's solution is blue in color, and if the test showed no sugar, it would stay blue. If there was sugar present in my urine, it would change color to designate a trace, 0.5 percent, 1 percent, or 2 percent.

My results were always supposed to be a trace to 1 percent. A few negatives were allowed, but no 2 percent were allowed. The testing was very inconvenient, but the doctors who were led by the AMA didn't care about the inconvenience; all they cared about was the lab accuracy of the tests. Trying to maintain a small amount of sugar in my urine and accomplish it by monitoring it with this idiotic test was both confusing and frustrating, like trying to walk a tightrope. So after a while I quit doing the test.

In the beginning of my diabetic care, my mother gave me my insulin shots. Back then there were no disposable syringes. The syringe had to be assembled before each shot and disassembled after each shot for sterilization purposes. The needle, which was metal and had to be twisted onto the syringe, was of a heavier gauge than the disposables that are used today, and they were more costly. The injections were uncomfortable, but because the needles were expensive, you tried to get as much use out of them as possible before throwing them away after they became quite dull. Because the shots were uncomfortable, I was willing to let my mother give me my shot each morning. It had its drawbacks though. Whereas I was willing to change doses as I saw fit, my mother wouldn't make any changes without the doctor's permission, and as she prepared the insulin syringe, I had no control over it.

This all led to a very big mistake I made with my diabetes. Because I couldn't stand screwing around with the Benedict's solution, I quit testing my urine and would phony up test results that would please the doctor. I also quit testing because it seemed my test results always wanted to be either negative or 2 percent and rarely be a trace or 1 percent. My test results were probably 20 percent negative, 20 percent at best that were what the doctor wanted (trace to 1 percent), and 50 percent to 60 percent at 2 percent. So when the doctor was shown the correct results, I wasn't following my diet properly, and I guess not properly regimenting my life according to him. One thing that everyone could not seem to understand was that if you're not getting any fun out of life, what the hell sense is there in living it? If you are getting any fun out of life, you sure aren't going to be able to maintain that idiotic trace-to-1-percent level. So I decided to show phony results and be free of arguing with the doctor about anything.

The only major problem was that with the phony results, the doctor did not see any need to increase my insulin. Although I told my mother I needed to, she listened to the doctor and went along with the doctor. My test results were now running constantly at 2 percent, and I should have come clean with my test results but felt all I would get was more crap about how I wasn't sticking to my diet and regimenting my life properly. But little did I know that I was drifting into a diabetic coma. I don't remember exactly when this happened, but it was about a year after being first diagnosed with diabetes.

I developed severe abdominal pain, so my mother called the doctor, who immediately came out and diagnosed that I was going into a diabetic coma and needed to immediately be admitted to the hospital. Instead of my mother sending me to the local hospital, she chose Boston Children's Hospital; she felt they would have better doctors, and new and better doctors would get me on the right track with my diabetes. I recovered quickly from the coma, but they kept me at the hospital for about five days, I believe. I don't know why they kept me; they made no changes except an increase in the dose. Maybe they wanted to observe how my diabetes was behaving. Well, life in a hospital is a lot different than home life. You're doing different things at home rather than living life in a test tube like you do in a hospital, and certainly once I got home, the dosage would have to come down because I would be more active.

Back then, the only kind of insulin I knew of was Iletin. The only instructions I received were to take twenty units every morning, and that was as far as any explanations went. No one explained what the duration of the insulin was or when it peaked in strength during the day—nothing. The only thing that was explained was insulin shock and what to do about it.

Now I was at Boston Children's Hospital, and my mother decided to have them supervise my diabetes. My mother took me to Boston once a month at first, I believe, then it went to longer durations later. One thing they did change, though, was the system I used to test the sugar being spilled in my urine. I believe the system was called Clinitest. This worked by measuring so much water and urine into a test tube and dropping a tablet in it. It would fizz up and change color, and that would designate how much sugar I was spilling, much the same as Benedict's. The only thing that was easier was that I didn't have to boil it for five minutes, but it was still lab accurate (big deal).

I didn't find these people to be any smarter than my family doctor. Questions that I asked about my diabetes remained unanswered. They just seemed to be more enthusiastic but gave me the same answers: nothing.

At my first return visit, they hardly said anything or paid much attention to me at all beyond telling us to make another appointment for next month. At the next meeting, they reviewed my urine test results again and noticed that they were erratic: more negatives and 2 percent than traces and 1 percent. This time there were two doctors in the room with me and my mother discussing the erratic control of my diabetes. All of a sudden, one turned to the other and said, "Do you think he is a good DBI candidate?" and then they abruptly left the room. The only thing that went through my mind was "What the hell is wrong with me now?" and my mother wondered the same thing. They didn't explain anything until they came back five to ten minutes later.

When they came back, they presented my mother with a bottle of a drug called DBI and said it would smooth out my diabetes control problems and that it would not behave so erratically. Now, why couldn't they have discussed this with us before leaving the room abruptly and leaving us to sit there and worry about what was going on?

We returned to Boston for a few more visits so they could see the results of the drug. There were no beneficial results from the drug, but they wanted me to keep taking it, along with the penicillin that our family doctor had prescribed over a year ago. They said I was doing better when I wasn't, but of course all they wanted to do was keep shoveling drugs down my throat. When my mother and I got home, I told her I wasn't interested in going back, and she reluctantly agreed. A month or two later, I took it upon myself to quit taking the DBI and the penicillin. Later my mother checked to see if either prescription needed to be refilled and noticed that they did not. She wanted to know why, so I told her I had quit taking them. Her response was that she didn't know what good either of them were doing me anyway. I would also like to mention that two or three years later, DBI was pulled from the market because it was creating too many problems for diabetics—even deaths. Guess I quit taking it none too soon.

I was fourteen years old and not interested in seeing any more doctors. They weren't doing me any good, so why waste my time? My mother was at a loss to know who to take me to, so she didn't push it. One problem, though, was my eyesight. It was consistently deteriorating. I needed stronger lenses with every visit to the optometrist. This bothered me, because at a recent visit to the public library, I had tried to find information on diabetes. Information about treatment was scarce, but one article I did find stated that better than 50 percent of diabetics were dead within twenty-five years after being diagnosed with diabetes, and a good percentage of the rest suffered from blindness, kidney problems, and other complications. I would have been willing to bet the small percentage without problems were the ones who turned their backs on the medical profession. Anyway, reading this didn't make me feel that my prospects for a long life were very good. It led me to believe that I would be lucky to live past the age of thirty-eight, and with my eyesight going the way it was going, I sure as hell would be blind. I didn't completely give up, but by the time I was seventeen, I had pretty much developed an attitude of live for today and the hell with tomorrow. Now don't think I had developed a death wish; no one ever has a death wish—they just decide to live life to the fullest and take what chances come their way, but that doesn't mean they have some jackass death wish. Hearing someone say that someone has a death wish has always irritated me.

At this time in my life, there were no blood tests to determine how good one's control of the disease was. Now we have the hemoglobin A1c test that determines how good your control of diabetes is. Back in the sixties, there was just urine analysis that determined how much you were spilling in your urine, and you were always supposed to be spilling some. I felt this wasn't getting me anywhere, and the test methods I was allowed to use were too inconvenient, so I quit using them, although not altogether. I tested infrequently just to keep an idea of what was going on. I would check myself if I felt I was not spilling any sugar to make sure that I wasn't. If I felt I was spilling a lot, I would check to see if I was. It helped me get in tune with my body and how it felt and what my urine levels were. Unfortunately, I should have paid closer attention to the negative readings, but the medical profession indoctrinated me to always run a trace. The funny thing about this method, though, was that I was finally running more traces than I ever had before. Don't forget, though, now I was able to control the amount of insulin as I saw fit.

At one time I asked a pharmacist if there were any more convenient ways to test my urine. His reply was "What does your doctor recommend?" and said that I had to go by doctor recommendations. I probably should have asked another pharmacist, but I didn't. It was like the doctors had a stranglehold on you and there was no way you could break loose from it.

The next five years went by uneventfully, except that by the time I was eighteen, I started drinking, and with each year more so. At the age of nineteen, I was out of school and working as a draftsman at a company I enjoyed working for. After a year with the same company, my drafting led me into quality control, and I became a quality control technician for the company. I don't want to get into my work history, but this bit of my work history is necessary to explain what happened when I reached twenty-three. I would like to end this part of my life by saying I started partying a lot and drinking a lot. The beer-drinking of these days raised hell with my diabetes and glucose levels, but hard liquor seemed to lower my glucose. There were times when I was out at clubs drinking and dancing when I would have to sit down and eat whatever snacks were put on the tables for the patrons because I was going into insulin shock. I was now twenty-two, and my life had turned to turmoil because the company I'd been working for had closed the division I worked in and moved it to Phoenix, Arizona. Only management people and engineers were transferred to Phoenix, and my boss and I were not among them. The company did talk to me and tried to encourage me to go to college. They said they could set me up with the financial aid to pay for it all and keep me employed at their other divisions on a part-time basis while going to college. I gave it serious thought and had the greatest of trust in the company, but I still didn't see a lengthy future for myself, so I turned them down. I was twenty-two, and four years in college would make me twenty-six at graduation. I would only have ten or twelve years to make use of a college degree. As you will see in the next chapter, it was a good decision medically speaking.

Chapter Two

Finally Free

After losing my job, I worked at two different jobs and wasn't happy with either. I left the first one, though I shouldn't have. I went to a second one and totally hated the company, but while at this job, I was approached by my old boss from my previous quality control job. He had taken a position as a quality control manager with a company that had a small division in Pennsylvania. He wanted me to relocate from Danielson, Connecticut, to Pennsylvania and help him set up a quality control system for the division, and I accepted the offer.

So I moved to Coatesville, Pennsylvania, because they had a YMCA where I could stay until I found an apartment. It was the end of July of 1969, a little over ten years since I first was diagnosed with diabetes. My eyes now required a lens strength of -6.00 in my left eye and -5.00 in my right eye. Overall I believe my health was declining also. In Connecticut I wasn't seeing a doctor and didn't plan on seeing one in Pennsylvania either. After all, they hadn't done anything for me before; why should I expect anything different now?

My boss had stuck his neck out for me in giving me this job because my license was under suspension in Connecticut for drunk driving, so he had to pick me up each morning and bring me to work with him. Coatesville was on his way to where we worked, so it wasn't much out of his way. I continued to drink, especially after work because my boss liked to stop at a local bar with others from work—not all the time, but occasionally.

Things were going well until around the end of November. I caught either a bad cold or the flu. I was still living at the YMCA, and they kept the temperature at barely sixty-five degrees. I had no way of keeping drinks in my room, and I kept my insulin in a refrigerator in the cafeteria, which was on the floor below. I didn't feel that this was an ideal situation to get over my illness. Since my license was under suspension, I called a cab and told him to take me to the Coatesville hospital. When I admitted myself at the hospital, they asked me who my doctor was, and of course I responded that I didn't have one. They then assigned me a doctor whose name was J. Deaver Alexander. Dr. Alexander and one other doctor are the only doctors I will mention by name because I have no respect for any of the others and may leave myself open to lawsuits by writing ill of them. But Dr. Alexander, I write kindly about and admire as a doctor. As far as I'm concerned, he saved my life.

He immediately took me off the Iletin insulin and put me on Lente insulin and regular insulin. He said there were two choices now in insulin: Lente and NPH. He felt that Lente was superior to NPH. Through the ensuing years, I found that he was absolutely right about Lente being superior to NPH. At times I couldn't get Lente and had to settle for NPH. Apparently a lot of doctors didn't prescribe Lente but instead went with NPH. Why did this occur? I can only speculate. The duration of Lente insulin is longer than NPH. Most doctors go by the recommendations of the AMA. Because of the longer duration of Lente, the control of my diabetes was better, and I'm sure it would have been likewise with most people. I don't believe the AMA ever wants to make anything easy for the patient but instead as difficult as possible, so they encourage the use of NPH—the same as the lab accuracy of Benedict's solution.

Next he put me on two shots a day of insulin: one in the morning, which included Lente mixed with regular, and a second shot before dinner. The second was a lesser amount than the first, and both were best taken an hour before my meal. Unlike the mealtime insulin of today, it takes more time to get coverage from regular insulin, so the shot had to be taken an hour before I ate. Before meeting Dr. Alexander, I didn't eat breakfast because my glucose would soar if I did. Dr. Alexander told me I wouldn't have to skip breakfast anymore. He also told me if I wanted to go out at night and drink and have fun, I should take a little regular insulin and enjoy myself.

This gave me new freedom with my life, but what really set me free was when I told him how I was testing my urine and was always supposed to be spilling a trace. He said to forget all that and joked about it. He gave me a plastic case with a roll of yellow litmus paper in it. It was called Tes-Tape. He said when you have to urinate, you pull off about an inch and pee on it. If you're spilling sugar, it will turn green; if you're not, it will stay yellow, and he also said he wanted me to have 80 percent to 90 percent negative (yellow). He said he would like all negatives, but he was afraid I would be having too many insulin reactions if I was controlling it that tightly. The amount I was spilling was meaningless to him. He said, "You're either spilling or you aren't. Shoot for negatives." Finally I was set free from the previous idiotic crap and given the means to actually control my diabetes.

While I was in the hospital, he regulated me on my new insulin regimen. After a few days, he had me leave the hospital in the afternoon because he wanted to see how some outdoor activity would affect me. After a few more days in the hospital, he said I was ready to go home, but he wanted to see me in a couple of weeks to see how I was doing. One thing he had in his office was a unit that measured blood glucose levels. We started to play a game with it, which I initiated by telling him what my glucose reading would be before he took my blood sample. He was amazed that I was always so close, usually within twenty points of the reading. After the first time, he would ask me what the glucose reading would be, I would tell him, and he would verify it. One time at his office, though, I felt I was on the verge of insulin shock. He checked my glucose, and it came up 120. We were both surprised. He thought about it and felt possibly before I became diabetic that my body controlled my glucose higher than normal, but there were other times when my glucose was at or near one hundred and I had no feeling of insulin shock. We came to no conclusion about why it happened. Now that I monitor my own glucose, I find it still happens, but infrequently.

I continued to see him every three months for the first year, but even though I liked him and enjoyed the visits, I felt every three months was overkill, so he let me change to every six months. I was doing really well with my diabetes to the point of trying to see how many days in a row I could go without spilling any sugar. Because now it was so simple to monitor myself, I would check with the Tes-Tape every time I had to urinate. I went as many as twenty days in a row without spilling. My diabetes was under great control. After three or four years with Dr. Alexander, I started to become lax in making my appointments with him. At one time I went a whole year without seeing him. When I did make the appointment and showed up at his office, he remarked about not having seen me for a year. The first thing he did was take a blood sample to check my glucose. After he got the result, he went out and loudly proclaimed to the nurse, "What do you think of this guy? I don't see him for a year, and his glucose is at one hundred." The control of my diabetes was so good that now every time I visited the optometrist, it was to get weaker lenses, and my eyesight stabilized at -3.00 in my left eye and 2.50 in my right eye—half the strength of the lenses I needed before. Dr. Alexander was one of a kind. Whenever I was at an appointment with him, my medical records were always where I had easy access to them. He felt they were as much my business as his, and if you ever had a question or something to say, he never tried to make you feel stupid about it or ignore you like many other doctors do. He never had an air of arrogance about him; he never had to feel superior to you. He only took adult patients because he said he wanted patients whom he could trust. I not only knew him professionally, but I got to know him personally. He was always willing to talk to me, at least to a degree; after all, he did have other patients.

Let me back up in this a little bit and give you a little bit of personal history that is important. I was twenty-three years old, and it was shortly before my twenty-fourth birthday that I met Dr. Alexander. I got married three and a half years later in 1973. As you already know, I drank heavily, and I also smoked heavily—a three-packs-of-cigarettes-a-day habit. When I got married, I quit both smoking and drinking.

Now that I was married, a problem arose that I had never had before. I was going into insulin shock at night, two times so severely my wife had to call an ambulance. Each time I woke up to see Dr. Alexander's face and the concern on it, but there wasn't anything he could do to prevent them. I was the only one who could do that, but it would be a few years before I could. See, I had no real idea where my glucose was before going to bed. Although I was pretty good at approximating what it was, it would play tricks on me. I would usually have a snack before going to bed, but sometimes I would forget or I would think it wasn't necessary because the previous morning I had woken up spilling sugar. Most of the time I would be so wound up in trying to keep a string of days free of spilling any sugar I would lose sight of the other problem.

The year was now 1977 or '78 (not sure which), and I had just started a new job as calibration lab manager at Exxon Office Systems. (Its original name was QYX.) Also, my wife and I had horses, and we would ride together frequently. We both had western saddles and English saddles—or, as Dr. Alexander called them, eastern saddles, and it is what I prefer to call them. Anyway, one weekend, my wife decided she wanted to ride western for a change because we both preferred eastern. I was into jumping and always liked to take my horse over at least a few jumps while I was riding him. So there were a few jumps set up, and I just had to take them. My horse was a good jumper but had a tendency to refuse jumps when things were different. As he approached the jump, he hesitated and then refused but in the last instant decided to take it. The only problem was that when he refused, he brought me forward over the horn of the saddle, and then when he decided to take it, he slammed the horn of the saddle into my ribcage. It hurt a great deal, but we took our ride anyway, although we cut it short because the real pain was beginning to set in.

The following day I made an appointment with Dr. Alexander, and I believe he took me the following day. He examined my sore rib and said he didn't believe it was broken, but it was probably cracked. He next said to go home and take it easy and let it heal. He also said it was unnecessary to x-ray it because even if it was broken, it would require the same treatment: rest. He also said that he could tape me up with wraps, but the only good that would do would be to make me feel as if he had done something for me. There were a few things he told me to try not to do and closed with saying, "Don't jump with a western saddle anymore." I guess I saw him on Monday and went back to work in the afternoon of the following day. It was summertime, and the sun was always shining. QYX was a startup operation and was spread out in small plants throughout the industrial park. I was in the process of inventorying equipment, and every time I had to leave my building, I would end up stepping out into bright sunlight. Anytime bright light hits my eyes, I sneeze. Needless to say, the next month with my ribs was hell for me every time I sneezed.

I don't remember if this was the last time I saw him. I may have seen him one more time before he retired. I don't know whether it was from a riding accident that he had when his horse went down on some ice, I believe, but he was having problems with his memory, and he felt he was not going to be able to adequately fulfill his duties as a doctor. I believe this occurred in 1978. I sorely missed him as my doctor.

Shortly after Dr. Alexander's retirement, in either 1979 or 1980, blood glucose monitoring was developed and put on the market for diabetics. I was still having a problem with insulin reactions at night and set out to find a new doctor, one who would introduce me to blood glucose monitoring. If I'd still had Dr. Alexander as my doctor, he would have immediately gotten me involved with it, but now I had to find someone else who would, and it was difficult.

I needed to find a new doctor. A person with whom I worked with recommended a doctor; he said his daughter, who was a nurse at one of the local hospitals, said this particular doctor was the best one at the hospital. So I made an appointment with this doctor with good expectations. At my first appointment, I explained what my problem was, which was insulin shock at night while sleeping. He said right off to eliminate the evening shot, which I did. My next appointment was a week later. The day after, an afternoon blood glucose test was done at the hospital. When he met with me, he didn't ask anything; he just said I was doing fine and to come back in another month. I responded by telling him the prior night, I had gone back to taking my evening shot. He got mad and told me not to make any changes, not even the amount of dosage, without his approval, and no evening shot. I told him that my glucose was way too high in the morning, and it made me feel sick. He said my glucose was returning to normal in the afternoon, so I was in control and that feeling sick was all in my head. This irritated me, and I told him, "The problem with you is you have nothing in your head." Needless to say, he was no longer my doctor. So much for recommendations.

This one was just a general practitioner, so I decided the next doctor would be in internal medicine. My fingers did the walking through the yellow pages, picked one in internal medicine, and made an appointment. When I met him, I told him my problem with nighttime insulin reactions, and this fool did nothing but shrug his shoulders. So I asked about blood glucose monitoring, and he said he didn't know anything about it. Now I was starting to get irritated and asked, "Do you know where I can find out something about it?" He told me one of the local hospitals held a diabetic clinic something like the first Monday of every month and that maybe they might know something about it. So I called the hospital and found out when they had the clinic and went to it.

The clinic was held in a conference room at the hospital. As I approached the room, I was met by a nurse, who asked if I needed help with anything. I said I was looking for the diabetic clinic, and she said she paid attention to the people who came to the clinic because most of them came on a regular basis for help and support, but I wasn't familiar to her. I told her that it was my first time and that I was looking to be familiarized with blood glucose monitoring. She immediately responded by telling me about what was available, which was BG Chemstrip. She said they can bought in a container that held fifty strips. She then said, "Don't tell anyone that I told you this, but you can cut them in half and then you will have a hundred test strips." I asked why she didn't want me to tell anyone, and she said, "Because I will get in trouble if it gets around that I tell patients how they can save a little money."

I wasn't going to stay for the clinic now that I had gotten what I wanted, which was the name of the test strips and how to use them, but I was there, so I decided to go in and see what went on. They had a doctor who got up in front and gave a talk. I don't remember what it was about, but I was a little impressed, so I decided that since I didn't presently have a doctor that I would give him a try. I called his office the following day and made an appointment with him.

At my first appointment, he wrote a prescription for the usual assortment of blood and urine tests and wanted me to keep a record of my blood glucose readings to give to him at my next appointment, which was in a month. At my next appointment, everything went well; he liked my blood glucose readings and all my other tests were fine. He said he was going to leave my dosages of insulin where they were and to come back in three months.

For those who aren't familiar with the first blood glucose monitoring device, let me explain. BG Chemstrips were plastic strips with material adhered to one end. The test material at the end was about three sixteenths of an inch square. You pricked your finger and squeezed a drop of blood onto that little square area. If you were using a meter, you had to cover the whole square with a drop of blood. Let me say it took a big drop of blood to cover that little square area, and I have seen nurses have trouble with these test strips. So by cutting the strips in half, you would need only half as much blood. Now, once you covered the test area with your blood, you had to wait one minute and then wipe the blood off, wait another minute, and insert it in your meter or compare it to the color chart on the side of the canister your strips came in. You paid about thirty-five dollars for a canister of fifty test strips, and after a month of using them cut in half, I said, "Why not start cutting them in three strips?" Now I had one hundred fifty test strips that cost me thirty-five dollars and required a lot less blood.

Now back to my new doctor and my third appointment with him. I sat down in his examination room, and the first thing that he asked was to see my blood glucose readings. The next thing he said was, "Why are all these readings ending in zero?"

I said, "Because when I compare the color of the test strip to the color chart on the canister, that is all the accuracy that I'm capable of and that I say is necessary."

He responded by saying, "You can't read them as accurately by comparing them to the color chart as you can with the meter."

I said, "Yes, I can," and he immediately had the nurse bring the meter over.

He got a test strip and said, "We will do a test where you can read it off the color chart and I will use the meter." He also said, "I will let you see the meter reading after you give me your reading from the color chart.

I said fine and gave him a drop of blood. After the test was complete, I compared the test strip to the chart and said my glucose reading was 120. He immediately turned the meter around and showed me a reading that was almost twenty points higher, and then we got into an argument. I told him my reading was more accurate than his meter and that he'd better get the damn thing calibrated. I told him to try looking at the chart. I was lucky with where the reading fell because the chart had a color sample right above the number 120. Sometimes your reading would fall between two color samples and you would have to decipher just where your test strip fell between the two. This one happened to match one of the color samples ideally. He had a hard job arguing, but he did anyway. Then he continued to say that I had to use the meter and that the meter came with a device that cut the test strips in half so that I wouldn't have to struggle with scissors. I knew this was an outright lie because the meter would only read whole test strips. I told him he was a liar and that this just showed how unreliable his meters were and that my readings off the color chart were more reliable. This got under his skin, and then I said, "You're not my doctor anymore," and left.

Chapter Three

Life without a Regular Doctor

For about the next sixteen years, I had no regular doctor. If I had a problem, I sought out a doctor and had the problem taken care of (if you can call it that). Usually I had to handle the problem myself, even with things other than my diabetes. I stopped letting doctors get involved with my diabetes entirely and had more than one argument with doctors over it. This chapter will show the outright incompetence of the medical profession. Excuse me, that is pretty much what I've done through the last two chapters, with the exception of Dr. J. Deaver Alexander. So this chapter will actually be more of the same.

My next experience occurred one day when I was exercising my horse by myself. He was shoeless and the ground was wet, making for a slippery situation on horseback. When I took my horse out of the pasture, I separated him from a mare of which he was a little too fond, and while we were in the rink, he kept being a handful, wanting to get back with his mare. He was a gelding, but sometimes he didn't act like one. Going around one corner of the rink, he slid on the wet ground and went down with me still straddling him. My foot was still in the stirrup, which got twisted around my foot from the weight of the horse. It must have hurt his ribs a great deal also, but he seemed fine. He got up, and I mounted him again and tried to keep riding, expecting to get him over some low jumps, but the pain was too much. I decided to quit riding and I took him to the barn, unsaddled him, and let him get back with his mare. I then drove home and got out of my riding gear and had a very difficult time getting my riding boots off.

When my wife got home, I told her she had to take me to the hospital because I thought my foot might be broken. She had gone shopping, so she put her things away, and then we got in the car and went to the hospital. I went to the emergency room, and after a brief wait (it was now late in the evening), I was taken into x-ray and my foot was x-rayed. I was then brought back out to the waiting room so I could wait for the results. I don't remember how long I waited, but eventually someone, an x-ray technician or a nurse, came out and told me there was nothing wrong with my foot and that it was just badly bruised, so I went home.

The following morning, the hospital called me and said my foot was broken and asked if I had any preference on a doctor to take care of the break. I said, "No, whomever you recommend will be fine." They set up an appointment for me that day, and my wife took me to it. When I got to the doctor's office, he was a young doctor, and he said that the bone was broken but not displaced, so all that was necessary was to put a cast on it. I asked to see the x-ray. He got out my x-ray and put it up on the viewing screen, and when I looked at it, I could see the break right away. I didn't even have to look closely. I told the doctor that they had sent me home the previous night after telling me there was no break, that it was just badly bruised. How could that be when the break was so obvious? He smiled and made a remark that I guess was somewhat condescending about the hospital staff that night and then put the cast on my foot. He then told me that I would have to keep the cast on for over a month, possibly six weeks. I gave him a date that was just before a weekend for which I wanted the cast off. The reason was that I was a white water kayaker and wanted to catch a local dam release out of Nockamixon State Park. The stream became a good run with the release, and I wanted to catch it. He said it would be too early, but we would wait and see. I do believe he told me to come back in a week or two weeks because the cast would need to be changed after the swelling in my foot went down.

When I saw him again, he removed the old cast and put a new one on. I made an appointment with him for the day I had previously specified, and I anxiously waited for that day. When it came, I went to his office again. He checked my foot and said it was fine, but he wanted to leave the cast on for another week. I told him I wanted it off. He said, "If you insist, I will take it off, but your foot will be so sore you're not going to be able to do any kayaking anyway."

He took the cast off, and he was right; it was sore, and I still needed crutches to get around. The morning of the dam release, it was still so sore all I could do was go to the release and watch others enjoy while I walked around on my crutches. The doctor was absolutely right, and I liked him. He took the time to get to know me and understand me. There was no air of superiority and the expectation that I had to do exactly as he said. He knew I wouldn't be able to use my foot, but he also understood what something meant to me and allowed me to find out for myself. I wish I could remember his name. I would have used his name in this book because my memory of him is with respect.

From 1981 to 1986 or 1987, I worked as a river guide on the Lehigh River, a class three river in northeastern Pennsylvania. I enjoyed the company that I worked for and most of the people with whom I was surrounded. The pay wasn't great, but I thoroughly enjoyed what I was doing. I almost always enjoyed the guests on the river. On some rare moments, I'd have a raft with some people who couldn't grasp rafting either out of fear or stupidity, and they would cause problems on the trip that would take away some fun from the others, but these occurrences were rare.

There were three levels of guides; class one were the only ones who could be trip leaders, and there were always three other guides on trips down the river. The other guides were usually level two and three. I started out as a level three and sometime during my second year became level one and a trip leader.

Let me now explain what this has to do with my diabetes. On raft trips I always carried a couple of rolls of Lifesavers (the candy) with me. They kept well and were easy to carry. I used them to combat insulin reactions, which happened too frequently. Although I took less insulin while guiding and it was quite a bit less, it wasn't always little enough, so I would eat some Lifesavers—sometimes it was both rolls. When the raft trip was over, the rafters were put on a bus and driven back to the campground, and before they got off the bus, I would get up and say how much we enjoyed having them as guests, then I would ask them how much they enjoyed their time with us. They always yelled and cheered loudly. Three or four times that I remember, I got up and must have looked like a complete jerk, and the people looked at me and wondered what was wrong with me. My glucose would be so low I would stutter and stammer like a complete idiot because I couldn't remember what to say. I couldn't muster any thoughts or anything else, and it would leave my guests surprised and wondering what was the matter. I never advertised that I was a diabetic back then. I would try to keep it to myself as much as possible, which led to these kinds of problems. I did at one time, which was rare for me, lean down to a woman on the bus and said, "I'm a diabetic, and my glucose is low. Do you have anything with sugar in it for me to eat or drink?" She didn't but immediately found something for me, and I thanked her. It averted one of my crises, but I was only on the verge of an insulin reaction and not into it yet; otherwise I wouldn't have asked. It is amazing the tricks diabetes plays on you and the tricks that are played on your mind when your glucose falls. Of course, your brain needs an adequate amount of sugar for it to function properly, therefore the mind tricks.

At this point in my life, my diabetes had regressed to the point of my insulin needs being as high as 120 units a day. While on the river, I would sometimes get cramps in my hands and arms, mostly at the beginning of the year when I was out of shape, but it would still persist on occasion throughout the year. To combat it, I decided to get into weightlifting. I had always exercised and kept myself in shape, but I felt I needed more, and weightlifting was the answer. It helped a great deal the first year. I started this my second year as a guide and kept increasing my effort in it, and I still work out with weights today.

My last two years as a guide, I started taking a packet of vitamins and amino acids that I bought from a nutritional store that was produced especially for weightlifters. I was already taking a multivitamin pill, but this packet was something new to me, and I wanted to improve my weightlifting ability, so I decided to give it a try.

It almost immediately increased how much I could bench-press, plus my overall performance. I was very happy with the results. Not only did it help me with the weightlifting, but with continued use of these packets of vitamins and amino acids, I had to start reducing my evening insulin shot. The packets did not include balanced amino acids. There were two primary amino acids and then low dosages of the essential amino acids—those that have to be consumed because the body does not produce them itself. The two primary amino acids were arginine and ornithine.

I continued taking these packets from September to the summer of the following year. I was lowering my evening insulin dosage a unit and sometimes two units each week to the point of not having to take the evening shot at all. Next, my morning shot started to lower to the point where I was down to under fifty units a day. My morning shot had also lowered during the disappearance of my evening shot, but not very significantly. Right now I bet any of you diabetics reading are saying, "What are those amino acids you're talking about? I want to take them." The next chapter explains the most tumultuous time in my diabetic history, which I believe was caused by the packets I was taking.

Chapter Four

Bouts with Monosodium Glutamate

I started taking the amino acids in the early fall of 1985 and continued through to the summer of 1986. The packets that I was taking were expensive, and the instructions on the box the packets came in said to take one packet daily, but I was working out every other day, so I decided to save some money by taking the packets only on the days I worked out. The effect I was getting was still good—in fact, excellent. By April of 1986, I was down to forty units of insulin a day and only one shot in the morning, and no evening shot was necessary.

By the middle of May, I noticed I was no longer getting any effect from the packets concerning my diabetes, but I kept taking them anyway. One other problem I was having was that every once in a while I would have a feeling of anxiety that was uncomfortable and a feeling of doom. These anxiety attacks were also accompanied by depression, and it all climaxed in the middle of July.

The second week of July, my wife and I took a week off to go camping at Allegheny National Forest in the northwest corner of Pennsylvania. I decided we would end the camping trip Saturday morning and drive down to Ohiopyle, Pennsylvania, to meet with some friends who were kayaking the Youghiogheny River, and I would enjoy a day of running the river with them on Sunday.

While on the river, I kept suffering from cramps in my arms and hands, and at times it was quite uncomfortable, but I enjoyed the day and the company anyway. After getting off the river, I loaded my kayak on my pickup, connected the camp trailer, and my wife and I headed home.

That evening, when we got home, I felt somewhat lousy, with a feeling of doom and some shortness of breath. I had had these feelings in the past two months three or four times, but this was a little bit worse. I chose to ignore it anyway and went to bed that night. I had a good night's sleep, but when I woke, I felt worse than the day before, and now I also had chest pains, so I told my wife to take me to the hospital because I thought I might be having a heart attack.

My wife took me to the hospital, and I was admitted. I will state the name of this hospital because I have nothing derogatory to say about them, and I therefore won't have to worry about a lawsuit. The hospital was Brandywine Hospital in Coatesville, Pennsylvania, and during admission, they of course asked what my problem was and who my personal physician was. I told them I felt as if I were about to die and that I had shortness of breath and some pain in my chest and also that I was not presently under the care of any physician. They agreed with me that I might be having a heart attack. I don't completely remember what happened next, like what tests were done and where they were done. When I say I don't remember, it's because I have been in the emergency room of hospitals more than a few times, and it gets confusing to recall what happened in each instance.

Next I was in the cardiac care room in the hospital (they hadn't assigned me a room yet), and they were doing an electrocardiogram on me. After the EKG was completed, I was approached by someone, possibly someone in administration, and he informed me that they were assigning a particular doctor to me. I didn't know him, and I rejected him, choosing to go with the doctor my wife had and liked. This was a very big mistake on my part. I should have accepted the one the hospital assigned. My wife's doctor turned out to be a complete moron and, as far as I was concerned, was not fit to be a doctor, as you will learn next.

The cardiologist who was assigned to me was the next one to present himself. He informed me that the blood that had been drawn had tested positive for a general muscle enzyme that shows up when you have had injury to your muscles and that he was waiting on the results of an enzyme test that is directly related to the heart but doesn't show up until twenty-four hours after the heart attack. I stayed in the cardiac care room the rest of the day and most of the next day.

I awoke the following morning about seven o'clock, and a nurse approached and asked what I wanted for breakfast. I don't remember having much of a choice, but I made some kind of a selection and then asked about my insulin shot. The nurse responded by saying it would be given to me in a short while. At eight o'clock, they brought me my breakfast but no insulin shot, so I asked again where my insulin shot was. The person who gave me the breakfast tray assured me I would receive it in a few minutes. Slightly annoyed, I decided to eat breakfast anyway. I always took my shot an hour before I ate; that way my breakfast was covered well and my glucose never rose that high, certainly never up around 200. But this doctor with a two-digit IQ wouldn't let them give me my shot without his approval. Finally somewhere around ten o'clock, they came in with my insulin shot. By now my glucose had soared, probably between 300 and 400, and I felt lousy, like I was getting sick. I complained to the nurse about the timing of my insulin shot, and she responded by saying it didn't matter when I got my shot as long as I took it at some time. I don't know what kind of nursing training this woman had or whether she was just following what the doctor told her. Quite frankly, I thought it was a lot of stupidity on the part of the nurse and doctor.

A short time later, the cardiologist came in and told me the enzyme directly related to the heart was negative, but they were still concerned because the general muscle enzyme was positive. So I made a vain attempt to explain that on Sunday I had been kayaking and suffered from cramps, and for a brief time they were severe. Wouldn't that be the reason why the general muscle enzyme was positive? What was most irritating was that they didn't even address what I told them. It was as if I had never spoken at all. As a patient, with many doctors, you're regarded as a dog in a lab experiment: be obedient, don't bark, don't growl, don't bite, and let them have their way with you.

Next they sent me to another floor in the hospital for some tests. They wheeled me around on one of those hospital beds used for transporting people when they want you to stay flat on your back because if you sit up, it is going to put too much stress on your heart. When I had rheumatic heart disease, I had to put up with the same kind of bullshit, and it makes me wonder if anyone in the medical profession has enough intelligence to understand how stressful it is to have to lie flat on your back and not be able to take in what is going on around you. It would be a lot more relaxing if the patient was allowed to sit up a bit, maybe not perfectly upright, but not flat on your back either, but what do I know? The medical profession always downgrades patients' intelligence to a few points higher than a dog.

I was transported down to a room where some tests were to be performed on me, and I was left out in the hallway until they were ready to do the tests. I was left in the hallway underneath an air conditioning vent in the ceiling that was blowing cold air directly down on me. I was quite cold lying there, and with my glucose somewhere over 300, I became sick. I tried and tried to get someone's attention, but to no avail. The bed had side restraints that prevented me from being able to help myself. I raised my voice for over a half hour trying to get someone's attention. Finally I yelled with profanity, and that finally got me some attention. I was finally moved away from the air conditioning vent and about fifteen minutes later brought into the room for the tests. I had lain in that hallway for at least a half hour, during which I wondered whether they had forgotten all about me.

After completion of the tests, I was moved back upstairs to the cardiac care room. After they analyzed the results of the tests, they finally decided it wasn't necessary to keep me in the cardiac care room, so they assigned me to a room. The room had a telephone in it, and I immediately called my wife and told her when she came over to bring my insulin, syringes, and my BG Chemstrips. I was not allowing them to have anything to do with my diabetes anymore. It was all too obvious that the doctor I'd chosen and the nurse assigned to me had no understanding of the disease diabetes.

My wife came to the hospital late that afternoon with everything I'd told her to bring. I immediately used a BG Chemstrip to find out how high my glucose was. I don't remember what it was, but it certainly was over 300, so I took a shot of regular insulin to bring it down close to 100. The time was somewhere around four to five o'clock, and regular insulin usually had a six-hour duration, so this shot of insulin would have been active until around 11:00 p.m. and would have peaked at about 6:00 or 7:00 p.m. So at about seven o'clock, I rechecked my glucose level and found that I needed a few more units of regular insulin in order for me to get my glucose where I wanted it, which was as close to 150 as possible but not below 120. I wanted it in this area because I knew that soon as it dropped below 200, I would be able to shake the damn cold they'd given me. One other problem I had was that I didn't know exactly what they'd given me that morning. They said it was the same as what I said I took at home. So I asked why they had to wait until ten o'clock in the morning to get approval from the doctor, which ended up throwing my diabetes out of whack.

I guess it was about 9:00 p.m. that I felt my glucose was starting to approach 200, because I was starting to feel a lot better. By now I was comfortable with the feeling that my glucose was going to be right where I wanted it to be in the morning when I woke up, so I tried to get some sleep. I finally got to sleep, only to be awakened by someone to draw blood. After the person drew the blood, I went back to sleep. In strange beds, I'm a light sleeper, and I was awakened again by the same nurse who had told me that morning it didn't matter when I took my shot as long as I took it. She had an IV unit with her, and she started to approach me with it. I immediately asked what the IV was for, and she replied that they were afraid I was going into insulin shock, so they were going to give glucose to me intravenously. I knew my glucose had not dropped below 200 yet, and it sure wasn't below 100. I wasn't by any means in danger of insulin shock. So I asked her where my glucose was, and she replied—and I remember distinctly—210. I told her at 210 I sure wasn't in any danger of insulin shock, and she wasn't hooking me up to it. She said, "Doctor's orders. We have to hook you up to it." I again told her no, she wasn't, and she again said, "Doctor's orders." Now this really irritated me because she wasn't going to back off from this stupidity on her part and on the part of this pathetically inept doctor. She insisted on hooking me up to this IV unit, which would have elevated my glucose back over 300 and made the cold that I was now getting over worse. So I exploded and told her to get the f—— out or I'd take the f—— unit and wrap it around her stupid f—— head. Now she finally grasped the situation with me and left. Having to respond to someone in this manner bothered me because she was the only good-looking nurse I had to look at.

The whole scenario when you take a good look at it is just so profoundly stupid on the part of the doctor that it's amazing that someone like him practices medicine. First off, you don't go into insulin shock until your glucose drops at least below 70. My glucose was at 210; how could I be going into insulin shock? Second, I had all my faculties about me, and even if he was justified in thinking I was going into insulin shock, why not just give me a glass of juice to drink? Of course, the IV unit would have cost more than a glass of juice, and doctors try their best to get as much of your money and the insurance money as they can get. It doesn't even have to be going into their pocket, just as long as it goes into someone's pocket that belongs to the medical profession. This is just an example of how most doctors are never concerned with your best interests—just their own, and in a distant second, with those of the rest of the medical profession. There are not enough bad things I can say about this doctor that I had, but choosing him was of my own doing. I had much regret about not accepting the doctor the hospital had designated. After all, when they were Coatesville Hospital and at a different location, and when I admitted myself and had no doctor, they assigned one to me who turned out to be the best doctor I've ever had, previously and since. This was the doctor I talked about in chapter two.

The following morning I awoke and checked my glucose. I don't recall what the reading was, but it was in the vicinity of 100. I was feeling great and completely over the cold I had received from lying under the air-conditioning vent the previous morning. (One other thing I would like to point out about the air conditioning vent was that the only protection I'd had from it was a thin hospital gown—no blanket.) Next a nurse came in to take a blood sample and gave me a sheet with choices for my meals for the day. I don't remember how they were going to handle my insulin shot—that is, whether I was going to have to wait until 10:00 a.m. again or whether they already had approval on a dosage. But it didn't matter because I told the nurse I now had my own insulin on hand and my doctor was no longer allowed to be involved with my diabetes. I also told her I was monitoring my diabetes myself and I wasn't in need of their help with it, but if they wished to do any monitoring of my diabetes themselves, they could feel free to do so. She then abruptly turned around and walked out, and an hour later I was brought in my breakfast. For the rest of my stay at the hospital, my diabetes was never mentioned, except when I left the hospital.

Later that day, I believe they did some more tests on me, and of course they had me on a heart monitor. Thursday, which was my fourth day there, I don't believe any tests were done, and I don't remember if I was ever allowed to get up and walk around. I believe they kept me till Friday afternoon because they wanted to see if the monitor would pick up any abnormalities because all their other tests had found nothing wrong. Finally, on Friday afternoon, they released me, and my esteemed doctor came in to talk to me. This would be his first conversation with me. He had come in one other time and said hello and that he had to leave but would come back in a few minutes but never did. Now he made an appearance and said they couldn't find anything wrong with me, and he told me I was controlling my diabetes too closely by keeping my glucose below 200 all the time. He went on to say that his glucose levels rose over 200 after he ate, and then he handed me a prescription that he and the cardiologist would like me to take. They also wanted me to go into the University of Pennsylvania Hospital for a coronary catheterization. They had already set up an appointment for me, but I could cancel it if I didn't want to go through with it.

I responded to my doctor by first letting him know he didn't know what he was talking about concerning diabetes. Next I asked, "If you can't find anything wrong with me, what the hell is this prescription supposed to correct?" Then I addressed the catheterization. I told them to inform the University Hospital that I would take care of my diabetes myself while there, that everyone had to agree with it, and I needed a day to think about it, and if I decided it wasn't necessary, I would cancel it through them. They immediately called the university, and they agreed. They wheeled me out of the hospital in a wheelchair to the front door, and then I got up and walked to the car with my wife and we drove home.

Through the eighties, I used to run a lot from May till the end of September. I would frequently run two miles, the first one as hard as I could while timing myself and the second one normally to catch my breath from the first one. By July, I would have my time down under five and a half minutes and be working on getting it under five minutes. I never had the dedication to achieve it though. The first thing I did the following morning home was to run my two miles, and I felt fine afterward. Next I decided to go through with the coronary catheterization; because I'd had rheumatic heart disease as a child, with a heart murmur, I wanted to see just how good of shape my heart was in.

Four or five days later, I was at the University of Pennsylvania Hospital. I was admitted in the morning, I believe, and was immediately assigned to a room. I don't remember if there was any preliminary testing that was done, but I do remember the man they put in the room with me. He came in late in the morning and was also a diabetic. He was there because most of his foot had turned black. The following morning I was prepped for the catheterization. I wasn't allowed breakfast, so I didn't need any insulin. They did inform me of what my glucose level was. I don't recall what it was, but it must have been around 120 because the guy in the other bed with the black foot said, "Wow, mine is always up around three hundred," and I just had to reply with "Yeah, I know—that's why your foot looks the way it does." I guess it was about 9:00 a.m. that they came and took me down for the catheterization.

They gave me a local anesthesia where they inserted the catheter, and I was awake for the whole thing. I could see everything that was going on and got to see what kind of shape my heart was in for myself. It looked great. It was perfectly clean, nothing wrong with it, and it was great to be able to see for myself. Sometime around 11:00 a.m. or noon, I was brought back to my room, and they asked me how much insulin and what mixture I wanted. I told them what I wanted, and they brought it in as I prescribed and they gave me my shot. After they gave me my shot, the guy in the bed next to me said he wouldn't have had the foggiest idea of how much insulin to take. I told him I didn't know what kind of doctor he had, but he couldn't be much of one, and he needed to dump him and start learning how to manage his diabetes himself or his complications were going to get much worse. After I spoke, I took a look at his foot, which was always left uncovered, I was amazed at how much of it was already cleared up with normal color restored. It was remarkable to me how quickly they improved his foot. After all, it was only a span of twenty-four to thirty-six hours.

A half hour to an hour later, they brought me lunch, which I ate, and they told me I could leave later in the afternoon. Sometime later in the afternoon, they checked my glucose and told me they hadn't agreed with my insulin dosage, but what I had taken had worked out well for me. Their honesty and openness impressed me. I got to discuss things with them and even disagreed with them on a few things. They treated me with respect and not like someone beneath them. I left that afternoon with a great deal of respect for the University of Pennsylvania Hospital.

Before all this happened, my insulin dosage had fallen to about forty units a day. During this episode, it kind of backlashed on me. My insulin dosages rose to a single shot of fifty-six units, and it stabilized at that amount. The rest of the summer went great. Every morning I took the exact same amount of insulin and never had to vary it. Insulin now was like a very minor crutch to me. My wife and I took a trip one weekend, and on the trip I had a desire for some ice cream, so we stopped and had ice cream. When I checked my glucose, it had no effect on it. It was like I didn't have to worry a whole lot about diet. This persisted all the way to June of the following year. If it would have continued through the rest of my life, I would have been a very happy person. My diabetes wasn't anything more than the inconvenience of starting each day with an insulin shot. The rest of the day was as if I weren't diabetic. It was nothing but great.

Then June hit. My insulin dosages started to increase, and by the time I got to the end of August, I was back to two shots a day for a grand total of 120 units a day. I felt that heart attack assimilation had been due to the amino acid packs I had been taking before, so I was apprehensive about taking them again, but I couldn't rest with taking so much insulin again and decided to take the amino acid packets again. This time I decided to take them every day, thinking that taking them every other day had created some instability. When I started them again, the reduction in my insulin dosages was faster, and by the time I reached May, I was down to thirty units a day, but I was having anxiety and feelings of doom. They were more frequent and stronger than what I had previously experienced two years before. By the end of May or the beginning of June, I quit taking the packets. I was down to about thirty units of insulin a day and again one shot a day. I was also periodically having anxiety attacks where I felt as if I were going to die coupled with shortness of breath. Shortly after the Fourth of July, it came to a climax. This time I had another attack far worse than the other one for which I had gone to the hospital. The previous one had only slightly mimicked a heart attack, but this one felt precisely like a heart attack. I had pains shoot up my left arm, sharp pains in my chest, my shortness of breath was more severe, and I felt lousy. It came on quickly but was preceded by a feeling of doom, and after a few minutes it was all gone, even the feeling of doom, so I tried to forget about it. This happened in the evening, so after it was over, about an hour later, I went to bed and slept well. In the morning when I woke up, it was to a severe feeling that I was about to die and an overall lousy feeling. I wanted to ignore it, but this time everything was so severe that after a while I decided to have my wife take me to a hospital—a different hospital.

I was admitted to the hospital, the same one I'd gone to when I broke my foot. I guess that wasn't really smart thinking. Anyway, at the hospital again I had no personal physician, so they had to assign me one. They assigned the same doctor to whom I had briefly gone and whom I described at the end of chapter two. He was flat-out a liar, arrogant, and incompetent. I rejected him as my doctor, but the hospital stuffed him down my throat anyway. The doctor was a diabetic specialist, so that was the reason they insisted on assigning him to me, but just because someone is a specialist doesn't mean he is competent at it, and he wasn't.

My first meeting with this jerk was to be confronted by him about the fact that I didn't want him as my doctor. I responded by saying, "No! I didn't want you as my doctor. I had you for a doctor before. I didn't like you then, and I still don't like you now." He had no response; he just turned and walked away. After that remark, if there had been any intelligence and integrity from both the doctor and the hospital, they would have assigned me a new doctor. This just exemplifies how little regard this hospital had for their patients. Not all hospitals have such little regard for their patients, but most do.

I don't remember much about my stay at this hospital except that it was only for three days, and at one time I was asked, I believe, by their cardiologist whether I'd had any previous attacks. I told the person about my experience two years earlier. The person responded by saying, "So this time you figured you'd try another hospital and see if you could get a different result." I don't remember the words exactly, but I do remember they were expressed with an air of sarcasm. The one thing I do remember well about my stay was the confrontations between me and the doctor assigned to me.

The following morning, a nurse came in with my insulin shot. Before she gave me the shot, she said the doctor had changed my dosage from what I had said I took, but if I wanted, she'd change it back. I asked what he'd changed it to, and she told me. It wasn't a very big change, and I told her it wouldn't make much difference, so go ahead and shoot me up. The nurse was completely on my side, and she told me she'd heard I didn't want him for my doctor. When a nurse shows disrespect in that way for a doctor, it speaks well for the doctor, don't you think?

Later that afternoon, the doctor came in and explained to me that he had altered my insulin dosage, but it hadn't made any difference. I told him I was aware of the change, and if he made any changes in the future, he needed to go over it with me and get my approval. He turned somewhat red in the face. Anyway, he was pissed and turned around and walked out. I had been there only one day so far. He had changed my insulin dosage and said it hadn't made any difference. Difference? What did he have to compare it to?

The following morning he was back in my room and said they couldn't find anything wrong with my heart. He went on to say that they were going to check me for a hiatal hernia. He also said that the feelings of doom didn't come first, the chest pain came first, and because I'd gotten some pain in my chest, I'd become afraid I was having a heart attack. I told him he didn't know what he was talking about, and no matter what I said was happening, he was going to reconfigure it to suit his purpose. Then I bluntly told him that I had no hiatal hernia. Like the moron he was, he said, "That's why we're going to test you: to find out." I told him there was not going to be any test; I had no hiatal hernia, and I was getting dressed and leaving. I then called my wife and told her to come and pick me up. By the time I was dressed and had my stuff together, I went to the nurses' desk, and they told me where to go next, I guess (I don't really remember), but I did leave the hospital and was back home that day.

After about a week, I received a bill from the doctor of three hundred dollars for my co-pay for his services as well as the same amount from the cardiologist. I ignored them both and never heard anything from the cardiologist again. The other doctor was a different story that eventually led to a collection agency. I responded to the collection agency by informing them of how inept he had been and that he'd done absolutely nothing for me, and for those reasons, I wasn't paying. They stopped, and he then went to another collection agency. I responded to them by sending a copy of the same letter I'd sent to the other agency and never heard anything more about it. If ever you're dissatisfied, do not pay. If you handle it as I have, you will not have to.

While at the hospital I felt good, no anxiety, no pains, no nothing—especially no answers. Within a few days, I started to have the anxiety attacks again. They started happening every day and after a week, they got worse. It was like waking up to a nightmare almost every day. I started keeping a record of the attacks by rating them each day: zero if I didn't have one, one if it was mild, and two if severe. There were not many zeroes that I recorded, but plenty of twos. A lot of days were like waking up to a nightmare, and I started believing this was my last summer on Earth. My recordings showed there were trends to the severity and mild periods. It also showed a parallel to my diabetes, which was also not behaving well through all this. My glucose always seemed to run higher when my nightmarish episodes were worse.

So I went to the yellow pages to try to find a doctor who might be able to help me. I found one that sounded promising. He was retiring but agreed to see me anyway. He was a grand person and spent what seemed like an hour talking to me. After I explained what was going on in my life with my diabetes and the amino acids and how they affected my diabetes, he told me he was unfamiliar with what I was talking about and recommended a prominent doctor in Philadelphia who might be able to help me. I thanked this doctor and was very appreciative of the long talk we'd had. When I went to his receptionist to pay for the visit, she informed me that the doctor had said there was no charge. Like I said, he was a grand person from the start of my visit to the end. Too bad he was retiring; I would have liked him as my regular doctor. This occurred sometime around October of 1988.

Sometime around November or the beginning of December, I made an appointment with this prominent doctor in Philadelphia. He was located on the fifth or sixth floor of a building on City Line Avenue near the

Schuylkill Expressway. I made a total of three appointments with him, and the first one was to explain what was happening to me with the anxiety attacks and other problems. He spent his time analyzing me as a diabetic, the foot examination and such. Next a nurse drew blood, and that was the end of this visit. Of course, he wanted to see me in two or maybe as long as four weeks, which I did.

At the next visit, which I believe was late in the afternoon, he spent his time having me do a few exercises and then checking my blood pressure and heart. After he was done, he said he was going to have my heart checked by some heart specialists with whom he was associated. I told him no, my heart already had been examined by heart specialists. He responded that he wanted people he knew to give another opinion, and I told him I already had two opinions, including a coronary catheterization, and there weren't going to be any more opinions concerning my heart. I also told him that my diabetes was unstable and that at times I felt my body was trying to control my diabetes on its own. I told him sometimes I had problems with it staying at 150, and it wouldn't come down; even after exercise, it would still be at 150, and sometimes I felt as if I was going into insulin shock with my glucose at 150. I also told him that sometimes in the evening I would feel like I was going into insulin shock, so I would check my glucose to make sure, and it would be very low, so I would drink some juice and then wait for it to take effect. It wouldn't have any effect after waiting fifteen minutes and sometimes as long as a half hour, so I would have another glass of juice—and a few times, three glasses of juice—before my glucose would rise. He said that in order for this to be happening, my pancreas would have to be producing insulin, and that would be impossible since I'd been a diabetic for the past thirty years. However, to prove me wrong and to prove that I didn't know what I was talking about, he said he would test me for C-peptides. The test results would be in at my next visit.

Before my next visit, my wife was listening to a radio station that she always listened to while she was at work. It was talk radio, and on one show in the afternoon, they had a Dr. Schwartz whom they interviewed. He had written a book called *In Bad Taste: The MSG Syndrome*, and in the interview, he talked about different reactions that people had to MSG. He said MSG, or monosodium glutamate, was in food as a flavor enhancer. He described some of the reactions people have with it, such as shortness of breath, heart irregularities, and many more. After listening to the interview with George Schwartz, MD, my wife took down the information I would need to order the book, which of course I did.

At my next visit, I immediately brought up the subject of MSG and asked if it might be what my problem was with the anxiety attacks, with which I was still coping. The doctor said he was having me do a twenty-four-hour urine test and the test would also determine if I had an allergy to MSG. Next we discussed my C-peptide test. C-peptides are present in a normal person whose pancreas is producing insulin. The reference range listed on the test result sheet was .5 to 3.0. My test result was .8, which was on the low side of the range. It was in the range, but he said it was too insignificant to pay any attention to it. The range of the test was .5 to 3.0, and my test result was .8. You don't have to have a medical degree to understand that there was some significance to the test result. I don't remember during what time of the afternoon the blood was drawn for the test, whether it was early afternoon or late afternoon. If it was early afternoon, it would have been shortly after lunch, in which case the test result should have been higher; if it was late afternoon, the test result would have been correct for a normal person without diabetes. Still, the test showed without a doubt that there was some functioning of my pancreas. I doubt whether it was functioning normally, but it was producing insulin. This sleazy doctor refused to discuss it though. However, much to my regret, I disclosed to this doctor everything I had been doing with my diabetes, including the amino acids I had been taking.

Whether he took any of the information I gave him and pursued studies on it behind my back, I don't know. This doctor seemed so sleazy to me that I would not put it past him. One thing you have to understand about the medical profession is that they do not want to have anything to do with anything you can buy in a health food store or nutritional supplement store. I, however, feel in many cases any organ in the human body can be restored with the proper vitamin and amino acid supplements, but no research will ever be done on nutritional supplements because the pharmaceutical industry will not allow it. I will discuss this in more depth in the conclusion of this book.

After leaving his office, I went to the local hospital with the prescription for the twenty-four-hour urine test. On the bottom of the prescription, I had the doctor write that the lab was to send the test results directly to me. The doctor did it grudgingly. The hospital lab took the prescription, handed me a plastic gallon container, and told me every time I urinated for a period of twenty-four hours, it had to be collected in the gallon container. They told me I could start the twenty-four-hour period anytime I wanted and I had to end it the same time the following day and bring the container back to them that day. I completed the collection and returned the jug to them. A few days later, the book on monosodium glutamate arrived in the mail. The book was very informative and described a doctor who stressed himself with MSG and experienced what he felt was a heart attack. Also, the book did not mention anything about any urine test or blood test that could determine if you were allergic to MSG; there was no test except to be stressed by it.

The information in the book was completely contradictory to what this highly prominent doctor in Philadelphia was telling me. After all, he'd said this twenty-four-hour urine test would determine if I was allergic to MSG. So I decided to try to give the doctor who wrote the book on MSG a telephone call. I located him in Santa Fe, New Mexico, and on my initial telephone call, I couldn't get ahold of Dr. Schwartz, but whoever did pick up the phone took my message, which was that I had some questions about MSG. I thought it would be some time before I would hear from him, if at all, but two days later he returned my call and said, "I understand you have some questions about monosodium glutamate." I told him yes, I did, that after reading his book I felt that the problems I was having were due to MSG and I was presently going to a doctor who said a twenty-four-hour urine test would determine if I was allergic to it. He responded by saying absolutely not, that no blood test or urine test would determine if I was allergic; there was no test except to be stressed by MSG. He then asked who my doctor was and said he would be glad to call him for me and get it straightened out. I gave him the name of my doctor, whom he immediately recognized, and he said he'd studied medicine under him when he was in Philadelphia. I told him thanks, but I would handle the problem with my doctor myself.

A few days later I received the test results from my urine test. It was a microalbuminuria albumin test. This test looks for an excretion rate higher than fifteen micrograms per minute; if it is higher, you are at high risk of kidney failure. It seems that all this doctor was interested in doing was finding that my kidneys were failing or about to fail. My test result was 3.6, so he failed all the way around. The first two visits I had with him were for tests on my kidneys also. They just kept getting more specific as we went along because in his wretched mind I had been a diabetic now for thirty years and therefore must have kidney problems. The hell with what any of my concerns were; he never addressed them at all.

Late that afternoon, I called the doctor's office and stated my name. When he got on the phone, the first thing out of his mouth was to gloriously inform me that I wasn't allergic to monosodium glutamate. I then asked in a contemptuous manner, "How can you say that when I've found out the only way you can determine if you're allergic to MSG is to be stressed by it?" He started to stutter, "B-b-b-but why worry about it? It's in everything." I told him no, it wasn't, and that I already had been eliminating it from my diet and was beginning to feel much better and that I didn't need his useless services anymore. I also told him not to send me any bills because I would not be paying them. He tried to tell me that I had to pay for his services, but before he finished, I hung up on him.

I believe I paid for the first visit but stopped after that. You see, since I was having these nightmarish anxiety attacks and all I was getting was being jerked around by the medical profession, I decided to not give them any insurance information and try to string them along as long as I could. The only test that was paid for through my insurance was the microalbuminuria test. The rest were all done through his office. The blood was drawn at his office and sent out to a lab of his choosing, and then I was billed by his office, which I hadn't been paying. I no longer remember how much the bill was, but it had to be over two hundred dollars. When they were not providing me with any results and their only goal was to take as much money from me as they could, why pay them? I may as well have just sent in a hundred dollars a month to him and not bothered to waste my time driving into Philadelphia. After all, I received the same results.

However, a week later, I received a bill from him. I responded to his bill by writing a letter to him complaining about his lies concerning MSG and how he hadn't addressed any of my other problems. He wrote me a letter back with another copy of the bill and told me that I was confused about what he was trying to accomplish with me. I promptly replied with a very brief letter that read: "You're either a liar or incompetent. Quite frankly, I think it's a whole lot of both." I never heard another word from him. No more bills, nothing. I kept the letters for a while just in case he sent a collection agency after me. I would have forwarded the copies of the letters to the collection agency. After the last letter I sent, I guess he decided to drop it. It was the only bit of intelligence this prominent doctor had shown me, and please detect the sarcasm intended when I refer to him as prominent.

The book *In Bad Taste* became invaluable to me over the next month. By viewing my own personal records and my eating habits, I began to realize how much MSG I was consuming and when. I started to correlate my eating with my records on when I had my worst anxiety attacks. There was almost a perfect correlation. So I eliminated eating at all the bad eating places I was frequenting while on business trips. They were mostly fast-food places. Next, my wife and I went through our pantry checking food labels for MSG and hydrolyzed vegetable protein. After a month, my wife and I had just about eliminated all the MSG in our home, and life was now back to normal for me. The book was so valuable because MSG is put into our food under many different names, but if you identify MSG and hydrolyzed vegetable protein, you can remove most of it from your diet. No more waking up to a nightmare, no more depression—I was feeling great. I never was big on fast-food places, but they did for a while have a place in my life due to my work in quality control. It was amazing just how much of it was in my diet due to work and home. At home, one thing I was big on was soup; when at home, every lunch included soup. Unfortunately, soup usually included MSG as one of its ingredients. The use of MSG has diminished since the book *In Bad Taste* was published, but it is still out there in our food, and I do occasionally eat at a fast-food establishment without problems. Because I have diminished my level of MSG, it is no longer a problem.

What irritates me the most about this whole episode in my life is that the medical profession didn't have a clue about it, and when my wife discovered that MSG might be my problem and I presented a highly respected doctor with the possibility of my problem being MSG, he outright lied. Let me repeat: he lied!

I don't exactly remember when this occurred, but it did happen sometime during the eighties: I was bitten by a tick, and it gave me what I diagnosed as Rocky Mountain spotted fever. I wanted a doctor who was familiar with tick-borne diseases and not just some run-of-the-mill doctor because I was aware of how reluctant the medical profession was to diagnose Rocky Mountain spotted fever. At this time there was a referral service advertised on television for people to call, and they said they would refer you to a doctor who would specifically fit your needs. So I called this referral service and said I needed a doctor familiar with tick-borne diseases. They gave me the names of three doctors. Two were board certified, and one wasn't. I chose between the two who were board certified and took the one who was closest to me. His office was less than mile away from me.

I made an appointment for the following morning, which was three days after the tick bite. When I got to the doctor's office, his first question was who was presently treating my diabetes. The first thing you do at the doctor's is fill out a form that includes questions about your medical history. I somewhat stupidly put down that I was diabetic, so it left me open to a lengthy argument. I answered his question by telling him my diabetes was in excellent hands: my own. He right off started with how dangerous diabetes was and how I had to be under the care of a doctor—his care. We must have argued for five to ten minutes about my diabetes, and during that time, I became convinced he knew nothing about the disease. What convinced me was when I told him that my A1C tests always were between 6 and 6.5, he tried to tell me it should be lower, in the low fives, because of me being on insulin. If I'd had it that low, I would have been in frequent insulin shock. Finally I told him there was no way he was treating my diabetes and to address the reason I was there, which was the tick bite. He looked at the tick bite, which had a big dark circle around it, and immediately diagnosed it as Lyme disease. I asked him about the red spots I had all over my body, my arms especially. He said they were flea bites, and I needed to have my dog checked for fleas. I said they were not flea bites but were from Rocky Mountain spotted fever. The doctor informed me that Rocky Mountain spotted fever occurs in the Rocky Mountains and very rarely along the East Coast, and that was why it was named after the Rockies. He also went on to say that if it was Rocky Mountain fever, I would be a whole lot sicker. I told him to wait until the afternoon and I would be a lot sicker, that in the evening and morning hours I felt as if I was getting better, but by afternoon I was again sick as hell and running a fever. Typical of doctors, he ignored everything I said and wrote me a prescription for an antibiotic for Lyme disease.

As soon as I left his office, I went to the public library and researched both diseases. The book on Rocky Mountain spotted fever said the disease was misnamed because it was much more prevalent on the eastern seaboard and rare in the Rockies. It also stated that the severity of it could be mild to life-threatening and that the arms and hands became covered with red spots and could also cover other parts of the body. All this contradicted what the doctor had said. Also, it said the incubation period for Rocky Mountain was zero to seven days, and when I looked up Lyme disease, its incubation time was stated as at least seven days. I had told the doctor that the tick bite had occurred three days before my visit with him. The book also said that Rocky Mountain goes into remission in the evening and then comes on strong in late morning through the afternoon. For both diseases, the same antibiotic was specified, so I was lucky there; I had the prescription filled, and within a few days I was back to normal. It is appalling, though, that you can't trust a doctor to diagnose anything properly.

In the mid-nineties, I got into the hardwood flooring business and was in a woman's home installing a floor. She had once been a nurse, so I told her my story about the red spots and everything except calling it Rocky Mountain spotted fever. Before even completing the whole story, she blurted out, "Classic Rocky Mountain spotted fever symptoms." This woman used to be a nurse and was a lot smarter than that incompetent doctor. I asked why she was no longer a nurse, and she said she had gotten sick of dealing with incompetent doctors and also added, "Heaven help you if you ever really get sick, because the medical profession won't."

Chapter Five

Trying to Find a Regular Doctor

My bouts with MSG ended in the beginning of 1989, in February to be exact. The rest of 1989 went fine with no problems and no doctors. Everything kept going fine until March 1991, when I started to have discomfort in my throat. The discomfort kept getting increasingly worse to the point where talking was beginning to bother me. Finally, in April, it was getting bad enough that I figured I'd give the medical profession another try. So I went to the yellow pages and found a doctor who was an endocrinologist. When I met the doctor, I found him to be a young doctor and fresh out of college. He had just bought his practice from the doctor who was retiring whom I had talked to and who'd recommended the doctor in Philadelphia to me. I explained what I had gone through with the doctor in Philadelphia. He told me that the Philadelphia doctor's practice was the first one he'd looked into buying but that he wanted too much.

He right off wanted to analyze me as a diabetic patient. I told him not to, that I wasn't there about my diabetes but concerning the soreness in my throat. So he converted his attention to my throat, first looking down it with a tongue depressor. I don't recall any of our conversation concerning my throat except that I asked about my thyroid gland. Next he felt my throat with his hands and said there was nothing wrong with it. I responded, "You can tell that by briefly feeling my throat?" I told him I wanted tests done on my thyroid gland and that would give me more confidence that there was nothing wrong with it. He wrote a prescription for tests on my thyroid gland and a hemoglobin A1C test. I guess he was hoping to find that my diabetes was all out of whack. On the prescription I told him to write that I would get a copy of the results also. He did, and I immediately went to the hospital, had the tests done, and went home. I didn't care for this doctor, especially his attitude. He didn't really seem to care about me in any way. When I left, I didn't pay him, and he got no insurance information either. The thyroid tests showed nothing wrong, and the A1C test was 6.5.

Over the next couple of months, I continued thinking about my throat and what to do about it because it was slowly getting worse. By the end of June I had convinced myself that my problem was with my immune system and that it was attacking my throat—maybe my larynx, seeing as talking was my biggest problem. Sometime in the 1980s, I read a book written by a Dr. Braverman called *The Healing Nutrients Within*. He described all the amino acids and their effects on the human body. In the book he wrote about threonine and how it is an immunostimulant that promotes growth of the thymus gland. The body also needs it to keep the immune system in check by preventing the immune system from attacking its own body. So I got some threonine and took a capsule in the morning when I got up and another one an hour before dinner. At this time, I was taking about thirty-five units of insulin a day and only one shot a day. Over the course of a few weeks, the pain in my throat started to disappear, and at the end of a month, the pain was all gone and I had an added benefit, which was the lowering of my insulin dosage to approximately twenty-five units a day. But as I continued with the threonine, I felt a backlash with it. My insulin dosage started to increase. I immediately quit taking the amino acid, and my dosage returned to approximately twenty-five units a day and there was no return of the throat discomfort. Again, I'd had to heal myself.

It was now 1992, and for the past three or four years, I had been renting a three- or four-acre pasture for my wife's and my two horses. There was a four-stall barn with the pasture. In November 1992, I decided to put a concrete floor in one of the stalls that I was using for miscellaneous reasons, and I was sick of the dust from the dirt floor. The cement truck could not back all the way to the barn, so I had to wheelbarrow the concrete into the barn. I thought I could do it all by myself, and I did, although the concrete truck operator did give me as much assistance as he could. At the end of the project, I found I had given myself a hernia.

After about three weeks, even though it wasn't causing me any discomfort, I decided to get it repaired. I don't remember how I made the choice, but I chose Dr. David Bradford as the surgeon to repair my hernia. He was a surgeon who fixed hernias the old way, without putting some kind of fabric in there; that method is supposed to help you heal faster, but I didn't want any artificial material in my body. Although remote, there was a possibility that my body could reject the fabric used. I knew there would be discomfort after the operation, and I didn't want to be second-guessing whether my body was rejecting the fabric. In preparation for the operation, my doctor wanted me to get a chest x-ray, for what I don't recall, but I had the chest x-ray anyway. When I went to the hospital for the x-ray, the doctor who gave me the x-ray said I'd chosen a really good doctor for the operation and went on to say that if he ever needed a hernia operation, Dr. Bradford would be his choice for his own operation.

The operation went fine. I went to the hospital in the morning and left the hospital in the afternoon with the hernia all repaired. Now, this was twenty-seven years ago, and all I ever heard about hernia operations was how painful they were, but the discomfort was not that bad. If I remember correctly, I believe I only took pain medicine for three or four days and quit taking it. I hadn't hesitated to have the operation in the first place because I knew it was inevitable that I was going to have to have it done, and I knew the sooner, the better. If untreated, I believe hernias keep getting worse, and then the discomfort from the operation would have been worse.

Another problem came to light during the tests I'd had done before the hernia operation. A blood test showed that my triglycerides only measured twenty-nine. I asked Dr. Bradford about it, and he said I would have to ask a general practitioner. So I found a general practitioner, and his response to the low triglyceride reading was the lower, the better. I then asked, "Why do they list a range of forty to one hundred sixty on the test results and flag my low reading of twenty-nine?" His response was that it didn't matter and not to worry about it. I was concerned about it and decided to go to the library and do my own research.

At the library, I found a manual on all the medical tests performed and what the test results meant. On many of the tests in the manual, there were other tests that were suggested to have done to follow up, because the out-of-range test result was, many times, indicative of more than one ailment. Low triglycerides, it stated, were rare and mainly caused by abetalipoproteinemia, and I don't believe it specified any other tests to be done. Next I looked up the disease in another medical book. The book didn't have much information except that the symptoms were retinal pigmentary degeneration and neuromuscular abnormalities, and its cause was hereditary. I was now at a standstill concerning my triglycerides. This present doctor wasn't concerned and could care less.

Finally I got on the internet and got more pertinent information from a website that was sponsored by, I believe, Johns Hopkins. The website gave a lot of causes of abetalipoproteinemia and went on to say you cure it by taking large amounts of vitamin E. The only thing that bothered me about the website was that they could have been more specific about the amount, but I decided that I would start at four hundred IU at breakfast, four hundred IU at lunch, and four hundred IU with my dinner and get my triglycerides rechecked. So I had the doctor write me a prescription to have some more blood work done so I could see what my triglycerides were. Now you're probably wondering, why not just get my triglycerides tested? Getting the complete basic package of blood work done was only about five to ten dollars more. This was a previous lesson I'd learned. When I had him write the prescription, I forgot to have him write on it that the lab was to send results to my home, and when the doctor received the results, I asked for a copy. He refused and I exploded. I got my copy, but it was from a very disgruntled doctor. The small minds of these doctors are unbelievable. You're supposed to go to their office and let them treat you like you're a dog in a lab experiment and let them have complete control over you. You're not allowed to oversee anything or undertake any responsibility for yourself. They act like, "How dare you think you can interpret the test results?" After all, they spent years in college learning how to interpret them. Unfortunately that is all most of them learned, and most of them didn't even learn that part of medicine well. The results are presented in such a simplistic way, I could give a sheet of paper with test results on it to a kid in grammar school and the kid would be able to tell what is out of whack. Besides, this doctor said very low triglycerides were no problem. Anyway, that was the last visit with that doctor. The test results said my triglycerides were at thirty-six, so I decided to double my vitamin E dosage to eight hundred at breakfast and keep it at four hundred at lunch and dinner.

At this point, I would like to explain something that I briefly talked about in my introduction. I got involved with trying to have a legislation passed so that I wouldn't ever again have to have arguments with doctors over copies of my test results. Sometime around November of 1991, I approached Joe Pitts, who was then my state representative, and asked if he could introduce a legislation that allowed me to directly request copies of my test results from labs that were doing the tests. I explained that presently the state health department forbade it. He immediately informed me that it would be difficult for him to do because the House of Representatives was controlled by the Democrats, and he was a Republican, but he agreed to give it a try. At first he seemed interested in the bill because he talked to a friend of his who owned a medical test lab and he was in favor of it, but a short while later his friend died, I believe from a heart attack, and after that he seemed to have little interest. One thing that Joe Pitts did for me was to introduce me to the head of the committee that the bill would have to begin with. At the meeting, I was expecting a discussion would take place, but this committee head got up and said, "I'm in a hurry. You've got one minute." It caught me completely by surprise, and I handled my one minute very badly. I blame Joe Pitts for not setting up an actual meeting, but he probably did his best. I don't remember the name of the committee head, but all I can say about him is that he was a blatant jerk. He didn't have a bit of respect for me and could've cared less about anything I had to say. However, while in front of the capitol building waiting to meet with Joe Pitts, I was approached by someone who was also a representative and a Democrat. He said he had never seen me before and wanted to know why I was there. I told him I was waiting to see Joe Pitts about the legislation I was interested in. He showed an interest and asked me some questions. I didn't take down his name, to my regret, and I'm not sure whether he got involved, but I do know a bill similar to the one I requested through Joe Pitts was introduced some time later. It was introduced by the Democrats.

Through redistricting and a change in my place of residence, I shuffled through two or three different representatives, and they were always Republicans—and I don't mean it in a demeaning way. The last representative that helped me on the bill was Curt Schroder, who pushed the chairman of the Health and Human Services Committee to act on the bill in February of 1996. He also informed me of the Democratic bill that had been introduced, which was not too different than the Republican bill. When it actually was finally passed I have no idea; it was sometime around the turn of the century, but it was passed, and now when you have any medical tests done in the state of Pennsylvania, the lab has to inform you that you have a right to the results being sent directly to you. I don't know how much credit I deserve for the passage of the bill, but I did get the ball rolling, and it pleases me a great deal that in a small way I was able to stick it to the doctors. To intelligent doctors the bill probably means little, but I know it bothers the many stupid ones—that is, only if they have enough brains to know about it. My own doctor didn't realize I didn't need him to know what my test results were. I consider this legislation very important because as a patient, it gives you the right to information (test results) that allows you to make informed decisions and to know what questions you should be asking your doctor and not be left at their mercy.

Now I had to find another doctor to find out if I finally had my triglycerides above forty. I found another doctor, a woman doctor in practice with her sister, another doctor. When I told her about my concern with my triglycerides, her response was the lower, the better, but this time I had copies from the books at the library. I handed her the copies, and she read the information. She was right up front and said she knew nothing about it. She also stated the only way to prove one way or the other about the abetalipoproteinemia was with an intestinal biopsy, which she didn't believe I would want or was necessary. She then said to have the standard test done and we would talk about it. I did like her honesty, and she didn't try to just brush it aside and look at dollar signs because I'm a diabetic. I liked her and would have kept her for a doctor, but she had this arrogant, irritating receptionist that I couldn't stand. She epitomized everything that is wrong with medical people and their patients. So before I did something to her that I would regret, I decided it would be best to find another doctor. I should have made the decision immediately and said something to the doctor about her, but I did a slow burn about the receptionist after leaving and later made the decision. When I got my test results, my triglycerides were thirty-nine. I then decided to increase my vitamin E to eight hundred three times a day.

This occurred in March 1996. Later that year, Eli Lilly Company came out with Humalog insulin, a fast-acting mealtime insulin that starts almost immediately after injection and peaks over a two-hour period and rapidly diminishes afterward. I felt this insulin was going to be great when I heard about it: no more having to wait an hour or two to eat breakfast after taking my shot. You never needed a prescription to buy insulin, but because Humalog was a new kind of insulin, the hierarchy of the medical world used it to tighten their hands around the throats of diabetics. You needed a prescription to buy Humalog insulin.

I didn't know this until I went to buy my first vial of Humalog. When I went to my usual pharmacy to get the insulin, they told me it was so new they hadn't received a shipment of it yet, so I called around, found a pharmacy that had Humalog insulin, drove to this new pharmacy, and asked for a vial of Humalog. The pharmacist went to the back and came back with a vial of Humalog and then said he needed to see a prescription. I told him you didn't need a prescription for insulin, and I said it in a threatening and very rude manner. He got scared and gave me the insulin without any more requests for a prescription.

I went home and the following morning started using the insulin, and it lived up to all my expectations. It gave me more freedom with my diabetes, and I would be willing to bet that the AMA was doing a slow burn over the development of this insulin because now diabetics would have better control over their diabetes. When I first started buying this insulin, it sold for about fifty dollars; now it sells for one hundred twenty dollars. The price more than doubled in fourteen years? I feel as if I'm being ripped off.

I continued going to the same pharmacy where I'd bought the first vial of Humalog and got away with buying the second bottle without a prescription, but on my third try, the owner of the pharmacy was there, and he said "Yeah, I've heard about you." He asked who my doctor was. I told him I didn't have one. He said he could understand why and went on to tell me that he could phony up a prescription with a doctor they used for such things, and he would enable me to continue to buy Humalog without a prescription. I knew it was illegal, but I didn't care. If I'd had to go to a doctor to get a prescription, I would have had to go through a lot of crap and wasted time. This continued for about two years until one day I went to the pharmacy for a vial of Humulin L (Lente), and they were closed with notices on the premises that the government had closed them. I guess the owner had had a far-reaching sale of drugs to other people set up in the same way as mine, and it had finally caught up with him. I was aware of what was going on, but I have so much contempt for the medical profession in this country that I happily ignored it. Now I was going to have to find a doctor and have to stick with him in order to get the insulin I needed.

I imagine that some of you readers have a bad impression of me from the last paragraph, but in my opinion, it was totally out of line and wrong to require a prescription for Humalog insulin. It is quicker-acting—so what? I don't know whether a prescription was ever required to purchase insulin. Insulin is so mandatory to a diabetic from day to day; you can't just say, "I can do without it for the day." Now suppose you go on a trip, let's say to California, and you arrive late in the afternoon, four or five o'clock. You get to your hotel room and the first thing you do is look for your Humalog insulin because you need it in order to eat, but it has been misplaced; probably, you forgot to pack it. Now it is eight or nine o'clock back east and you're going to go through hell trying to get your Humalog replaced—all because the hierarchy of the medical world has decided they don't give a damn about you but are concerned with giving as much control over your life as they possibly can to the doctors. When insulin was first being used to treat diabetes, problems such as the one I just described were either foreseen or experienced, and it was decided that prescriptions should not be required for the purchase of insulin. I believe at one time, years back, the medical profession had a genuine interest in the welfare of the public they served, but in today's world, they absolutely don't give a damn. The only thing that they cared about is control, control, control! Control of you and me, and not for our benefit, but theirs.

Now I needed to find a doctor before my Humalog insulin ran out. I talked to a woman who lived a few houses up from my wife and me and told her my predicament. She recommended her doctor and told me a little bit about him. I felt he was worth a try, so I made an appointment with him. When I met him, I told him it had been a while since I had seen a doctor and that I needed my prescription for Humalog insulin renewed. He then gave me the usual diabetic exam and wrote a prescription for the usual blood and urine tests for diabetics, and he also wrote me my prescription for Humalog insulin. I was always proud of the fact that I put myself on Humalog and was never supervised by the medical profession once in the use of it.

This visit was in January 1999, and now I could buy my Humalog insulin legally. It was by no means a big deal to me. This new doctor also wrote on the prescription for the blood and urine tests that it was all right to send the results to my home. Of course I had to tell him to, and he resisted a bit but complied. When I received the results, my triglycerides were at forty-nine. My A1c test was 6.7—a bit high when my A1c tests in the past were always below 6.5, but at least I now had my triglycerides within the test range.

My next visit with this doctor was three months later. I don't know why I allowed that, but I kept the appointment and allowed him to play the role of doctor. At this time I was still at thirty to thirty-five units of insulin per day. The previous doctor I'd had, the woman, was seemingly intrigued by how much insulin I was taking and made a remark about how low it was for someone who had been a diabetic as long as I had. This doctor, like all the others, had no curiosity about it, so I asked, "Don't you find it interesting that I take such a small amount of insulin?" His response was that what was more interesting was that I had been a diabetic for forty years and the test results showed no kidney problems. It seemed that every doctor I went to was expecting and a few, it seemed, actually outright hoped that I was either having or developing kidney problems. This doctor seemed happily amazed that I didn't, but his remark still irritated me a bit nonetheless. Let me give a little diabetic background. During the 1990s, a study was done on whether tight control or loose control was better. Loose control was where you were always spilling varying amounts of sugar in your urine because they had the belief that a glucose level of 200 was fine and necessary. Some doctors thought this was erroneous thinking, and so they decided to do a study to determine which control is best. The study determined that tight control was better and would prevent the typical diabetes-related problems. Now ask yourself, what kind of medical experts who drive the rest of the medical world could possibly think that elevated glucose levels would not be detrimental to your health? That moronic thinking that persisted until the nineties boggles my mind. The study showed conclusively that the closer you keep your glucose levels to the human body's normal level (70–110), the healthier you will be with diabetes. Of course you have to be more cautious of insulin shock. This will explain the next part of my conversation with this doctor.

When he said I had no signs of kidney problems, I responded by telling him about Dr. Alexander and that he'd had me on tight control since the beginning of 1970. He then replied that he must have been a doctor way before his time, and I replied, "No! He just had something the rest of you don't." Like a fool, he asked what that was, and I just couldn't resist; I said, "A functioning brain in his head." He didn't even seem to be insulted by the remark; he just went on about business as usual and ended the appointment with a prescription for the usual tests.

My next appointment was fifteen months later. I kept going to this doctor once a year until November of 2005. During this period, my cholesterol usually ran about 180, and at one appointment he tried to get me on statin drugs because he said diabetics' cholesterol should be below 150. I told him my cholesterol was fine right where it was. He tried to reiterate, and I stopped him by bluntly saying it was fine where it was. He didn't like the exchange, but I didn't need an unnecessary drug forced on me. I will expand on this in my conclusion.

At my next appointment, which was eighteen months later, we had a confrontation about my blood pressure, which five years previously always was 120 over 80, which was ideal. But over the course of five years, it crept up to 140 over 70, which is still acceptable but kind of borderline. It became an issue, though, because when she took my blood pressure, the nurse said it was 150 over 70. So the doctor was going to make an issue out of it, and I told him he had better instruct his nurse on how to take blood pressure so that she comes up with the proper reading. This fired him up a bit, and he wanted to know how I was so sure my blood pressure was not at 150, so I told him that I could read the meter and I could feel when my pulse started and what the pressure was at that instant, and my high was 140 and not 150. He didn't double-check my blood pressure but still tried to convince me to consider blood pressure medicine. I told him I would try to control it naturally, but I wasn't taking any blood pressure medicine. One thing I have to say to his credit is that concerning my cholesterol, he did suggest policosanol to lower it. I was already using it at the time, and it hadn't lowered my cholesterol; in fact, it had raised it by raising my HDL (which was a good thing because HDL is your good cholesterol), but when it raised my good cholesterol, it also raised my overall cholesterol reading because it had no effect on lowering my bad cholesterol. My cholesterol readings had been 180 and were now 200 with the elevated HDL (good cholesterol).

My last visit with this doctor was November 2005. At this time, as in the few previous years, I also needed a prescription for blood glucose monitoring. I don't remember exactly when it happened, but BG Chemstrips were no longer in the market. New brands were coming out that required less blood and had to be used with a meter because doctors all insisted that the patients were too stupid to interpret from a color chart. When it happened that I couldn't buy Chemstrips anymore, it made me angry. With BG Chemstrips, I was cutting the strips up into three strips and needed about the same amount of blood as all the new testing strips. I also paid thirty-five dollars for fifty test strips. That gave me one hundred fifty tests for thirty-five dollars, or twenty-three cents a test. The new test strips all cost about seventy dollars for a hundred at the beginning of the new century, or seventy cents a test. Now because testing had become so expensive, I started buying them by prescription so that insurance would pay for most of it. Before, I had never bothered with insurance or prescriptions. Presently it costs one dollar per test. The only advantage the new ones have is that BG Chemstrips required two minutes to complete the test, whereas it takes seconds with the new ones.

One problem I started to develop around 2003 or '04 was morning syndrome. My glucose would start to rise around four or five in the morning, and it would be 200 to 250 when I awoke in the morning. I used to take Lente insulin, which is now called Humulin L. While using Lente insulin, I had no problem with morning syndrome, but because the AMA directed doctors to prescribe NPH insulin instead of Lente, which was superior to NPH, the Lente became scarce, and it was frequently out of stock at the pharmacies and would have to be special ordered if I wanted and needed it. I decided to not put up with the bullshit and changed to NPH, known as Humulin N today. My problem was caused by the duration of the insulin. Lente had a longer active duration, which made it easier to control your diabetes over the day. The NPH insulin had a duration of about three hours longer than regular, which has a duration of six to eight hours depending on the individual. So if I took my shot at five thirty, an hour before I ate dinner, it would last till four thirty in the morning. Its duration was a bit shorter for me, leaving me with no insulin coverage after four in the morning. Both insulin start out as regular insulin but have a suspension added that impedes their absorption into the body. NPH suspension is different from the suspension in Lente.

At my last appointment with my doctor in November 2005, I asked about Lantus insulin, which is a long-acting insulin that reaches a level very rapidly after injection and maintains that same level for the entire day. My doctor said he didn't like long-acting insulin, or something to that effect. Whatever—I wasn't going to get any Lantus insulin from him or learn anything from him about it, so I decided it was time to find a new doctor. My A1c test was at 7.0 in 2003 because of the problem with morning syndrome, and in the next two years, I got my A1c test back down to 6.4 for both years. Why this happened was because every night, when the NPH insulin had dissipated and my glucose would start to rise, I would awaken and stay awake. The only way I could get back to sleep was to get up and take two units of Humalog insulin. I would go back to bed after taking the insulin and go right to sleep. When I tried to explain any of this to the doctor, I got nowhere. He seemed confused when I mentioned morning syndrome and didn't even understand what I was talking about.

Sometime during the winter at the end of 2005, I broke my femur while pruning my peach tree. In my back yard, I have a peach tree, an apple tree, and a pear tree. I also have raspberry bushes and a strawberry patch. I have this small orchard because I like to have a few months out of the year that I can eat fruit that hasn't been saturated with insecticide sprays. My raspberries and strawberries are never sprayed, nor are my pear tree or peach tree. The apple tree is the only one that I spray, but it is done minimally. I only get to eat the fruit when it's in season, but my berries are collected and frozen, and I eat them all year round. The raspberries, especially—I eat them on my breakfast cereal almost every morning. I also plant a vegetable garden, and that never gets sprayed. Two things I enjoy eating are fresh vegetables and especially fresh fruit. From the beginning of June to the end of September, they're my main snack. My wife and I have created a very friendly environment for birds, and during their nesting season, which usually isn't over till the end of July, my vegetable garden and raspberries go pretty much unscathed by insects. I didn't write this book to talk about organic gardening, so let me get back to my broken leg.

During the winter, I have to prune my three fruit trees. I used a stepladder to accomplish the task, one that was ill-suited for the job. I kept saying I needed to replace it but never did until after this happened. I had the stepladder upright under the peach tree with my pruning shears and was reaching to prune a branch. I reached too far and was too high up on the stepladder. The ladder went one way and I went straight down, landing on the ground on my hip. I lay there for a while and then slowly stood up. I was in a lot of pain but managed to limp to my house and got myself over to my easy chair, sat down on it, and relaxed. It was painful, but I felt that all I'd done was badly bruise it. My wife came home from work a few hours later, and I told her what had happened. She wasn't alarmed and went about preparing dinner. When dinner was ready, I managed to get up out of my easy chair (it was a recliner) and got myself to the table to eat. After we ate, I got up and went back and sat down to watch television. I had already resigned myself to the fact that it was going to be where I spent the evening: in front of the television. I spent the night watching television, and every time I had to get up for anything, it was a painful ordeal. I had my wife wait on me most of the time, but I'm just not the kind of person who can stay stationary for too long, plus I didn't realize yet it was broken. I went to bed that evening and tried to sleep, but I couldn't. I was in too much discomfort, so I eventually got up and went and sat on my easy chair and reclined and tried to get to sleep on the chair with a blanket over me. I think I got a little bit of sleep, but I know it wasn't much. The next morning I got up to relieve myself in the bathroom. I was expecting that the pain would be starting to subside, but it wasn't. I made it to the bathroom, and on the way back, I ever so slightly twisted my leg. When I sat back down in the chair and reclined, I looked at my feet and was surprised at the sight. The toes of my right foot were pointing at ninety degrees from where they should be. So I had my wife call the doctor. It was early in the morning, but we got ahold of the doctor anyway through an emergency number they give you when you're calling in off hours.

When we got connected to the doctor, I told him that I believed I had broken my femur and that I need to go to the hospital. He said he would make the arrangements and to go to the hospital, the one he was associated with. My wife drove me to the hospital, and when we got there, there was some confusion because they had the admission papers, but no one seemed to know where I was supposed to go. Finally a man came to me and said he was taking charge and got me to where I was supposed to go. He had me put on a gurney and a short time later wheeled me down to x-ray.

They took their x-rays, and I didn't even bother to ask about them because I already knew what they would find: my femur was broken. Plus all they would have said is "The doctor will talk to you about it." Because from the minute you're admitted, you're supposed to just lie there, shut your mouth, and let them have their way with you. While I was waiting for an orthopedic doctor to come and talk to me, I got a call from my doctor. This call was unbelievable. He started out, with his voice raised, and said, "You've broken your leg and you have to let them fix it, or you'll never be able to walk again." Then he repeated, "You've got to stay there and let them fix it." I cut him off by saying, "Who the hell asked to come here in the first place? Of course they're going to fix it."

A short time later, I was wheeled up to another area, and I lay there for a while. Finally an orthopedic surgeon came in to talk to me and said the break was four or five inches below my hip. He recommended a complete hip replacement but said I may be able to get away with just having it put back in place and screwed together. I asked what kind of restrictions on exercise I would have with the hip replacement. He asked what kind of exercise I did now, and I told him I presently leg pressed three hundred pounds and asked if I would be able to continue that. He said no, and I said, "Screw it together—no hip replacement." He seemed set on a hip replacement though because he continued by saying that once they opened my leg up, they may not have any choice. I then asked what the x-rays were for if he didn't know now what needed to be done. Finally he agreed on the screws, and I then asked to talk to the anesthesiologist. I talked to him for a brief moment and asked about the anesthesia, his experience with it, and when he had started this particular day. Everything was satisfactory to me, so I gave my approval for them to cut my leg open and screw the bone together. There wasn't really any other choice but to sign the consent forms.

Late in the afternoon I awoke and was in excruciating pain. Before even going to the hospital, I had packed my blood glucose monitoring equipment and my own insulin. While at the hospital, my glucose level was at 200 after the operation, and the following morning it was still a little above 200, but they had never once said a thing to me about my diabetes. It was as if they had absolutely no concern that my glucose was at 200. After I got my senses about me, I got my diabetes under control, and I don't ever remember anyone talking to me about it. The night after the operation and the first day, the pain was almost unbearable. I kept getting doses of morphine every three or four hours because it was the only way I could get any rest or sleep. That day I didn't do anything but lie in bed and get cared for by the nurses. The first day my leg was repaired, the second day was for recovery, and the third day I no longer needed the morphine, and sometime in the afternoon, I was fitted with crutches and I had to work with a physical therapist on how to use them. This was a bit irritating because crutches take a little getting used to, and any little misstep the therapist would blow out of proportion, as if she was trying to justify herself being there. That evening they started me on a drug called Coumadin. When they gave it to me, they kept selling it as a blood thinner, but I found out later it was actually an anticoagulant. At bedtime that evening, when they took my blood pressure, it was 160. I have no recollection of what the other half of the reading was.

The following morning or early afternoon, I was released from the hospital and went home. On the way home, my wife stopped to fill both prescriptions they gave me when I left the hospital. One was pain medicine and the other was Coumadin. I read the paper you get with prescriptions that tells you all you need to know about what the drug reacts with and whatever else you need to know about it. After reading the sheet on Coumadin, I decided I wasn't taking it. It not only raised my blood pressure but threw my diabetes out of whack also.

The following day a nurse was scheduled to visit and a physical therapist also. The nurse was scheduled to determine the level of Coumadin I needed to take, if I needed more or less. When she arrived, I told her she wasn't needed because I was not taking the Coumadin. I told her that they had given me one in the hospital and that stupidly I'd taken another one the night before, but I was not taking any more. She said that was fine with her and asked if I had told my doctor. I told her that I hadn't, but I intended to. She stayed a little while, though, and talked to me about my diabetes and said she was a diabetic also. She asked me if I used my fingers or my arms to get blood to check my glucose. I told her I used my fingers, that I felt my arms had too much hair on them and that I was comfortable using my fingers. She said she still used her fingers and asked if I used my little finger. I said no, that I was always told the only fingers you could use were your ring finger or your middle finger, and I had never questioned it. She then said that she used her little finger and would rather use her little finger, that it was the most comfortable to use. After our conversation, I started pricking my little finger for blood for my glucose check and found she was absolutely right.

Next the physical therapist came. I was right up-front with her and told her I wasn't in need of any physical therapy. She didn't dispute that but asked if I had taken a shower yet. I said no, but I intended to that night. She then asked if I knew how to get in the shower. I thought about it for a minute and said no, I didn't, so she proceeded to show me. I don't remember any other things she showed me but how to get in and out of a shower with crutches, but that impressed me. In my bathrooms, the shower and bathtub are ones with glass sliding doors with no way of sitting down on the edge and swinging your legs around, so I had to step over the bathtub to get in. It's funny how you get so used to doing something that you fail to see how you have to alter your approach and movement. I would like to think I would have figured it out by myself, but I don't know. All I can say is I had some resistance to her being able to show me anything, but she was very helpful. I enjoyed both the physical therapist and the nurse that day. Both of these people had the ability to talk to you and be personable with you, something few doctors are. Their arrogance always seems to get in the way.

That evening I quit taking the pain medicine and got a fairly good night's sleep without it. Late in the morning, I called the doctor who had fixed my leg and informed him that I was not taking the Coumadin. He said, "You've got to. Don't you realize the danger you're putting yourself in?" and then he asked why I'd stopped taking it. So I told him that it elevated my blood pressure and affected my diabetes. He responded that all that was caused by the pain medicine I was taking. I asked, "How can you say that when I'm not taking any pain medicine?" "You're not?" was his response, with a long pause. It gave me the opening to easily butt in, and I told him, "I'm still in a bit of discomfort but not enough that I need to take pain medicine. I have always been and still am a very active person and therefore don't need your Coumadin." He went on to try to convince me of the danger I was putting myself in. We had a bit of an exchange about it, but it was concluded that there was not going to be any Coumadin taken by me.

This doctor had outright lied to me when he said the pain medicine was raising my blood pressure and affecting my diabetes. Lies from doctors especially burn me up, but what also burns me is when they try to prescribe a dangerous and unnecessary drug. The reason to give a person Coumadin is if they're sitting or lying down and get up, they're going to break a blood clot loose and it is going to be carried to the brain or heart and it will kill them. I know I'd just had my leg opened up and a bone put back together, but I felt other things had to be considered rather than prescribing dangerous drugs needlessly. I also believe vitamin E supplements are a more suitable approach than Coumadin. I say this from my own experiences. I only take four hundred IU of vitamin E now because when I was taking eight hundred and I would check my glucose, I frequently had trouble stopping it from continuing to seep blood. When I reduced my vitamin E amount to four hundred IU, there was no longer a problem. All I had to do was wipe my finger once and there was no more blood. Does vitamin E have anticoagulant properties? I don't know and will never be able to find out from the medical profession, but from my own experience and an article I once read about vitamin E, I would have to say yes. Anyway, I increased my vitamin E amount during this period just in case there was anything to this bit about clots. Another point is if there are blood clots that might break loose, wouldn't it be better to do something about dissolving them in the first place? An anticoagulant prevents a clot from happening, but there was nothing I could find about Coumadin that said it dissolves clots that are already there. One thing I did find in a book concerning Coumadin was a statement that enlightened doctors called it killer Coumadin"

About three weeks after my femur was screwed together, I was still on crutches. I was getting up from the dinner table, and one of my dogs (we had two) was sitting near me and drooling in anticipation of her dinner. We have hardwood floors in our home, and my dog left a small puddle of drool on the floor that I didn't notice, and when I got up from the table, I put my right crutch in the drool and it slipped out from me, causing me to come down on my right leg, the broken one.

A week later, I was back at the doctor for a follow-up on how my leg was doing. My leg was of course x-rayed, and the head of the screws that were put in my leg were no longer flush with the bone but protruding out from the bone. They said my leg had collapsed and that it happens. I then told them what had happened with my dog, and they said that could probably explain it. I was then given another appointment; I can't recall what the time lapse was, and I'm not even sure that this appointment was at a month. It may have been sooner, but the slip I took because of my dog did precede it.

At this appointment I was again x-rayed. The doctor came in the room I was sitting in, looked at my x-ray, and went through a real effort to say my leg was still collapsing. After wasting my time and his own, he finally gave up and I left. This doctor was beginning to seem a bit sleazy to me. I do believe this was my three-month follow-up, because after this appointment, I didn't bother with any more follow-ups. I no longer had any trust in this doctor. He'd lied from the outset concerning Coumadin, and at this visit, he was really intent on trying to say my leg was still collapsing, when I saw the x-ray myself and compared it to the previous one, which happened to be present. There was no collapsing going on, and I'm suspect that the first collapse even occurred. I never got to see a picture of my leg immediately after the operation, even though I had asked, and I feel the screws may have been intentionally left that way. There was just too much concern about the collapse. The first notice of collapse was by a different doctor, and he was the one who said it does happen, but the one who did the operation was the one who kept making a big deal of it. I don't know what the motivation was except maybe he was still trying to get that full hip replacement. I still have discomfort in my leg, but I'm doing fine with it. The discomfort is minor and has more to do with my muscle, particularly where my leg was cut open so they could put the screws in. Whenever my muscle gets cut up, it seems to take a long time for it to get back to normal. I put up with the same thing with my hernia operation. I put up with minor discomforts for three to four years after the hernia operation.

Sometime toward the end of summer, I guess it was, I got a call from my doctor's office for me to make an appointment because they hadn't seen me for close to two years. I had been dragging my feet about finding another doctor, so I felt what the heck; I needed prescriptions refilled, and it would give me an opportunity to let him know what I thought of him. I wanted to do that face-to-face. One other complaint I had with him and his associates was that while I was in the hospital, the only recognition I got from them was when one day one of his associates stood in the doorway of my room, introduced herself, and then left. I had heard nothing from his office since. My biggest complaint that I wanted to rip him apart on was when he talked to me like I was a moron, and even though I'd had a broken leg, he thought I was going to leave it untreated and just leave the hospital. I had already diagnosed that my leg was broken, and I was the one who requested admission to the hospital. I guess it was because I refused to let him push statin and blood pressure medicine on me. My blood pressure is still 140 over 70 and my cholesterol is just below 200, and I would like to assure the whole medical world it is fine where it is. I don't need your drugs to correct it.

The appointment was made, and I appeared at it. I spent at least a half hour waiting just to get out of the reception room. I don't recall what their reason for the delay was, but there was no one else in the reception area, no patients when I arrived, and none came later. Finally over a half hour later, I was finally taken back to an examination room. After a few minutes, a nurse came in and asked me if I could give them a urine sample so they could check how much sugar I was spilling in my urine. I told her that I wasn't and had no urine to spill and that urine analysis for sugar went out with the introduction of blood glucose monitoring. I sat there for another ten minutes or more without anyone coming in to even weigh me or take my blood pressure, so I got up and left. I didn't really want to because I did have some things to say to him, and although I wasn't in urgent need of prescriptions needing to be refilled, I would be eventually.

Next I decided to immediately find a new doctor for prescription renewal and because I also wanted to try Lantus insulin since I was having a problem with morning syndrome (high glucose readings in the morning when I got up). I went to a few doctors and immediately determined they weren't for me, and the feeling was mutual. At the outset of the appointments, the doctors would ask why I was there or something to that effect. I would reply by telling them that I was a diabetic and under very good control—my own control, and it was going to stay under my control. One doctor was a woman doctor and said she didn't treat diabetes. One said he didn't treat people who insist on treating themselves. I said to him, "Oh, you like patients that come in and let you have your way with them? Well, no thanks," and I left. I got nowhere with these doctors and paid them nothing.

Finally, I made an appointment with one whom I liked, and it just so happened that he'd practiced with Dr. Alexander at the beginning of his career; he showed me a reflex mallet that he had with Dr. Alexander's name inscribed on the side of it. Now, just because someone was once linked to a doctor that I admired and respected didn't mean he would be of the same caliber, but I was sick of looking for an ideal doctor, especially when they're so rare to begin with, and this one seemed pretty good. He wasn't overbearing and wasn't a control freak. During this first appointment, which was in October 2007, we talked a bit about Dr. Alexander, and he informed me that Dr. Alexander had just recently died, that his obituary was in the paper. I must have missed it. It also surprised me to hear he'd recently died because the nurse that I'd threatened with the IV unit in the hospital when I experienced my first MSG attack had told me then that Dr. Alexander had died when I asked her about him. This had been twenty years earlier and before the IV unit incident. I asked about him because I would have liked to have contacted him just out of respect for him and to let him know how well I was doing with my diabetes due to him. It never happened due to the callous answer of that nurse.

Next I asked him about Lantus insulin, as I was having problems with morning syndrome and I felt Lantus might be my answer. He immediately stood up and left, returned with a bottle of Lantus insulin, handed it to me, and said, "Run it around the block and see what you think." I asked what dosage he recommended. He took a look at how much insulin I was taking and said to start at ten units at bedtime and adjust from there. He also went on about some sliding scale with my Humalog insulin in which I wasn't interested, and I paid little attention to what he said about it. I had already made up my mind on the insulin regimen to which I was going to adhere, and it was contradictory to what he wanted me to do. What the doctor wanted me to do was take the Lantus in the evening and use the Humalog all day long to maintain my glucose balance. That meant at lunch I would have to take a shot of Humalog, and if I wanted a snack, I would have to take some Humalog.

I decided I would take the Lantus in the evening in hopes that it would eliminate the high glucose readings in the morning and would supplement my usual insulin regimen during the day. My typical insulin regimen was Humulin N and a small amount of Humalog in the morning to handle the glucose from my breakfast. By continuing taking the N, I could continue my snacks in the morning and have lunch without needing a dose of Humalog, and I was also frequently in need of a snack in the afternoon. It gave me perfect control. My A1c tests were consistently below 6.5, and in both 2009 and 2010, they were 6.3. If you're wondering why I'm only giving the results of one test per year, it is because I only see my doctor once a year and sometimes it is eighteen months between visits.

I don't need to frequently visit doctors, and to their dismay, I refuse to. The only reason I see them at all is for prescription renewals. I maintain good control over my diabetes, and the yearly A1c test is only for reassurance that I'm doing as well as I think I am. Now if I would have let the doctor have his way with his insulin regimen, I would need to carry my insulin and syringe with me while working because I would need a shot of Humalog at least for lunch, and I would probably not be able to have any snacks. My regimen at this time was ten units of Lantus at bedtime, which allowed me to awaken in the morning with my glucose usually between 70 and 120. Once in a while I would screw up and it would be higher, but never over 160. Once I was up in the morning, I would take eight to ten units of Humulin N and four to six units of Humalog insulin. The amount depended on what my glucose level was when I got up in the morning. My next insulin shot would be before dinner when I got home from work. This shot was of Humalog and was usually four units but sometimes as high as six. It depended on what I was eating for dinner. If it was fish, all I ever needed was four units, unless my wife breaded it. Also, sometimes after work, when I got home, my glucose would be a little high, 160 or 180, and I would need a few units more. I could usually feel when it was high and sometime it would be over 200, but rarely. To determine if it was over 200, I would check my urine to see if I was spilling sugar in it. If I was, I would then check my blood glucose to determine just how much more insulin I would have to take. One unit of insulin would usually drop my glucose reading by fifty points.

Whenever it was over 200, it would be because my diabetes would deceive me into thinking my glucose was low and that I needed something to eat, so I would have a snack that I didn't need. What I felt was happening was my liver pushing glucose into my bloodstream to falsely keep my glucose high. It would feel like I was going into insulin shock when I wasn't.

When I started realizing this was happening to me frequently, I paid closer attention and detected a difference and could detect whether it was a real insulin reaction or a false one. These false insulin reactions had been occurring with me over the past ten years—maybe longer—and they kept getting more frequent and more severe. It seemed that my liver was trying to elevate my glucose over 200 at times. It was a problem for me if at bedtime my glucose was below 100 because I would need to drink some juice to elevate it. If I took so much as a small mouthful, my glucose would soar over 200 by the next morning. If it was at 100, sleep was impossible. I would have to either get up and take a small mouthful of juice or take a single unit of Humalog insulin. Either way, it affected me in a way with which I was not comfortable. If I took the insulin, my glucose would be fifty in the morning. If I took the juice, it would soar over 200 in the night, but I would have a sound sleep. Ideally, I needed my glucose at 120 to 140. I would then take two or three units more of Lantus to bring my glucose down to 100 in the morning. This effect kept getting worse the older I got.

This problem I was having came on so gradually. I thought it was just a problem with aging. I never asked any doctors about it; after all, I never got any answers from them concerning any of my problems before, and when I mentioned morning syndrome, my previous doctor didn't even know what I was talking about. So I developed an attitude that with my diabetes, I was all by myself. Another reason I didn't ask anyone was because I already knew what the answer would be from reading about morning syndrome. Most doctors will say to ignore it, and many of those won't even know what you're talking about. Contrary to the general opinion to ignore, it bothers me anytime my glucose rises above 200, whether briefly or, most of all, when it is constant, but every time I was in a hospital, no one was ever concerned about my glucose being at 200 and slightly higher. It was of no concern to them, even when I broke my leg in 2005 when it was already determined that tight control was better than allowing your glucose to remain high at 200 or above. Nevertheless, this problem kept getting worse and was very annoying to me until my eyes were opened by a problem with my medical insurance company.

My medical insurance would no longer pay for Humalog insulin and Lantus insulin. I was to convert to NovoLog in place of Humalog and Levemir in place of Lantus. I also had to visit my doctor and get new prescriptions for these replacement insulin. This irritated me; why should I need a new prescription if they were the same insulin as the others, just different manufacturers? After all, pharmacists prescribe generic drugs in place of name brands all the time unless the prescription is specific to deny any changes. Most of all and first of all, where does an insurance company get off dictating what insulin I must use?

My last appointment was slightly over a year before, so I was overdue—way overdue by doctors' standards, but I don't live my life by their standards. So I made an appointment, and when I got to the doctor's office, he was not there. He was held up at the hospital, and no one could give me an answer as to how long. So those present thought I should just sit there with my thumbs up my butt and wait indefinitely. Every time I asked, they could care less about giving me an answer, and I finally got irritated to the point of expressing my irritation verbally and left. I still needed the new insulin, so I had to make another appointment, but when I made the appointment, I told them I needed a bottle of the Levemir insulin now, that I couldn't wait for the appointment, so they told me that they had a bottle of it and that I could come in and pick it up, which I did.

When I got home with the bottle of Levemir insulin, I immediately opened the box the insulin vial comes in so I could read the papers in the box that you get with the insulin. I had been told by my doctor that it was the same as Lantus. When I'd asked a pharmacist, he'd said it was long-lasting like Lantus. So when I took a look at the papers that came with the insulin, I was slightly irritated to find out there were significant differences between Lantus and Levemir. Lantus insulin's strength peaks rapidly and its strength is flat or maintained at that level for its duration of twenty-four hours. Levemir is different because its strength rises at the outset a little more slowly than Lantus but peaks at a higher level for about eight hours and then gradually tapers off to nothing at the end of twenty-four hours. If I took it at night, I had to take a significantly lower amount, and I couldn't take it in the morning because it tapered off to almost nothing from three to six in the morning, when I needed insulin coverage. Another problem with the insulin was that the paper stated that the insulin inhibited the liver from releasing glucose into the bloodstream. This I did not want, but I was now out of the Lantus and had to take the Levemir. I felt I would only be taking it for a few days until a new prescription for Lantus was written. What harm could it cause in that short period of time?

This all occurred in June and July of 2010. At this time, I was up to twelve units of Lantus insulin at night. I decided to take only ten units of the Levemir insulin the first night I used it. The following morning I awoke, and when I checked my glucose, it was at fifty or sixty. The following night I took eight units, and in the morning my glucose was back to ninety. That evening I dropped it to another unit to seven units. Right now you're probably wondering what could be wrong with this since I was taking less insulin, but I wasn't taking less because I had to increase my morning dosage and my dinnertime dosage also. So overall, I was taking the same amount of insulin.

Next I ran out of Humalog a little before expected, so I had to call the doctor's office for a bottle of NovoLog insulin. They had a bottle of it and said I could come in and get it. When I arrived for the bottle of insulin, I asked to briefly speak to the doctor, that I had one question to ask. He came to the front, and I asked him if there was any difference between NovoLog and Humalog because there was a difference between Lantus and Levemir, and I was not happy with the Levemir. He replied they were the same: they were both quick-acting insulin.

I went home with the insulin, opened the box, pulled out the paper that described the insulin, and found that the insulin behaved much the same as Humalog insulin did but stated the same thing as the Levemir insulin did: it inhibited the liver from releasing glucose. This bothered me because I don't like any organs in my body to have their normal function altered. Also, this particular function was important to me and my particular lifestyle. For couch slugs who don't do much of anything, that feature of these two insulin was probably good, but for me and my active lifestyle, which included swimming in my pool and bicycle riding, it was detrimental. I took the Levemir insulin for only three days and the NovoLog for about a week until my insurance consented to allow me to continue with Humalog after my doctor had to assure them that I couldn't switch insulin. He did this because I gave him no choice, and it irritated me to no end that I had to put up with this from my medical insurance. It bothers me that you have to stand up to people in an abrasive manner to have the insulin and whatever else is right for you.

I imagine some of you are saying at this point, "What an arrogant son of a bitch. You're no doctor. Where do you get off thinking you know better than them?" Well, the summer of 2010 was an awfully hot summer, and I spent a lot of time in my pool. When I'm in my pool, I spend at least the first fifteen minutes actively swimming on top of the water and under the water. I swim the equivalent of a football field every time as fast as I can, usually in about two minutes or less. Then I dive three or four times, swim underwater, and then spend the next ten minutes or so swimming leisurely. After swimming, I would lie on my raft and soak up some sun. At the end of every summer, I would have a deep dark tan, but back to my swimming. The first time I went into my pool after taking these new insulin (they weren't new, but new to me), I didn't check my glucose before entering the pool. This was the beginning of July, and I had been swimming in June with no problems concerning glucose levels, but when I got done swimming my usual fifteen-minute routine, my glucose felt low, so I got out of the pool, dried myself off, and went inside to check my glucose. I wanted to make sure it wasn't a false feeling. Although I snacked before going into the pool as I normally did, my glucose was below fifty. From then on, I had to monitor my glucose before going in the pool and after I got out. Every time I checked my glucose after using my pool, it was always around fifty, even when it was as high as 200 before going in.

This was because, I believe, my liver was not releasing glucose back into my system like it normally should have. It was surprising to me because I'd never felt the effect would be that pronounced and linger for two months, especially after using the NovoLog and Levemir so briefly. It wasn't till the middle of August that the effect began to dissipate, and by the end of August, it had just about disappeared. The whole summer I didn't bike ride because I was worried about my glucose crashing while away from home, but in September, I took a bicycle ride of about fifteen miles, and while on the steepest part of a long, steep hill, my glucose crashed. When I ride, I pride myself on taking any hill that comes along and never walking up them. This hill was one of my favorites on which to prove myself, and here I was walking up the steepest part of it while eating a nutrition bar. What bothers me about all this was that the doctors have absolutely no knowledge that this problem exists with these insulin and are incapable of warning you about it. Like I said before, with this disease you're in it all by yourself. The medical profession has little help to offer.

This problem was generated by the medical insurance business Keystone Health Plan, a division of Blue Cross Blue Shield, to be specific. They meddled with my insulin medication, where they had no business. I was now annoyed at this meddling, so I decided to eliminate the opportunity for anyone to stick their nose into my treatment by taking advantage of my need for insulin prescriptions. Before there were any engineered insulin such as NovoLog, Humalog, Lantus, and Levemir, there was no need for prescriptions and no huge price for them. All four of these insulin cost about $120 a vial, and you need a prescription to buy them. For what? Sure, there are differences in both long-lasting insulin and the two mealtime insulin, but who cares? The doctors sure don't care. They don't even understand they're different. When Humalog first came out fourteen years ago, I paid around fifty dollars for it. Now it costs $120. These prices I have been quoting are prices that existed in 2010. The prices of these insulin are now close to $200. I don't have anything to do with any of them anymore, so I don't really know what the price is. Now I know Eli Lilly and Novo Nordisk, the producers of these engineered insulin, can come up with some outrageous and probably even sad stories of why they had to so drastically escalate the price of these insulin, but I will have the same answer to any of their stories: bullshit. Especially since Humulin N and R insulin still cost about fifty dollars a vial, a bit higher than what they cost fourteen years ago, but not more than twice as much. I don't buy anything in a pharmacy anymore, and I think they escalated their prices for the N and R insulin to $65 a bottle.

Because of price and the need for prescriptions, I decided to first eliminate the use of Levemir or Lantus insulin. You see, you kind of get in certain mind-sets, and they're not a good thing. Before, when I was taking Lente insulin, I could take both the Lente and regular insulin at the same time, which was an hour before I ate, and because the duration of Lente was longer than NPH, I had coverage through the night. But then Lente dwindled from use because of the AMA, and three or ten years back, production of it stopped completely. The one they should have stopped production of was the inferior NPH. The AMA knew this, and that is why they encouraged doctors to prescribe NPH. I wasn't getting the coverage from the NPH from 3:00 a.m. till dawn. I had a mind-set of taking the insulin before dinnertime because I really didn't want to have to take a third shot later at night. The Lantus broke me of that mind-set. You can't mix Lantus with other insulin. So I had to take a third shot with the Lantus. It broke my mind-set, because now I realized, why not replace the Lantus with the NPH at bedtime? I should have the coverage that I needed into the morning hours. This occurred sometime in July of 2010. Right after, I decided that Levemir was not for me. The first night I used the Humulin N, I decided on ten units, two less than what I was taking of the Lantus. The next morning my glucose was a little high, so the next evening I upped it to twelve units, and by the time August was over, my diabetes had regressed to the point of needing sixteen units at night. This was the regression factor that I have discussed previously in this book—that during the summer months, my diabetes regresses on me. Once I get into September, my insulin dosages come back down. Taking the Humulin N was keeping my glucose at one hundred most every morning I woke up.

Next I decided to eliminate the quick-acting or mealtime insulin. While writing this book, I learned one very important thing: I had thought I had been on Humalog since the beginning of the nineties, but when I called the Eli Lilly Company to find out for sure when I started using Humalog, they told me that they put it on the market in 1996. It surprised me because I had thought I had been on it since 1990. It started me thinking. I have always had an easy time with my diabetes, except for putting up with the stupidity and arrogance of doctors, but the past few years, it has become more and more of a problem. I never before had a problem with morning syndrome, and after thinking about it a lot since NovoLog was forced on me by my insurance, I'm beginning to believe it was a blessing. If NovoLog can hinder the liver from releasing glucose, why can't Humalog have the opposite effect? Maybe it forces the liver to release glucose.

Not only did I have morning syndrome, but also when I worked with weights, I would try to keep my glucose at 150 before starting my workout, which would last an hour. When I would get done and check where my glucose was, it would almost always be twenty to forty points higher than what it was before my workout. Also, after bike riding, my glucose would be higher than it was before I started my ride, except when I rode over twenty miles, in which case I would have to snack to complete my ride. If I did have to snack, my glucose would often be as high as 180 when I was done. My snacks were always 120-calorie nutrition bars, and I would only have one. I was also having constant problems with false insulin reactions. I would feel like my glucose was low, but when I would check it, it would be 140 or 150 and sometimes over 200. This was a real pain in the butt because I would feel like I needed something to eat, but if I did eat, sometimes my glucose would soar over 200, sometimes as high as 300. My kidneys were also being affected. At times when I felt like I was having an insulin reaction, I would check my urine for sugar to see if it was pushing my glucose level over 200, which it did occasionally. Twice when I checked my urine for sugar, it was negative, so then I would check my blood glucose to see at what level it was screwing with me this time. Once it was at 260, and another time it was at 240, but there was no sugar in my urine. I double-checked my glucose both times with different test strips with a different meter and got close to the same results, about ten points different. I probably should have checked my urine a while later. It may have been a delay in the sugar showing in my urine and would have shown up if I would have checked it later.

All this started out as a small problem some time ago and kept getting worse. The more I thought about it and after reviewing my records, I now believe that this problem started approximately twelve years ago, a few years after I started taking Humalog insulin, and this is the reason why I believe Humalog has the opposite effect that NovoLog has. NovoLog is up-front about it by disclosing the effect in the papers that they stick in the box with their insulin. Novo Nordisk states that NovoLog binds to the insulin receptors on muscle and fat cells and lowers blood glucose by facilitating the cellular uptake of glucose and simultaneously inhibiting the output of glucose from the liver. This is probably a good thing for those that never exert themselves, but for me it was a bad thing because I'm very active. If your liver is inhibited from releasing glucose when your body needs it because of exercise, your glucose crashes. Because of insulin and extended exercise, when not careful, this happens anyway, but with NovoLog, it sped up the process of my glucose falling, especially after switching immediately from Humalog to NovoLog. I have gotten rid of the Humalog insulin but kept a bottle of the NovoLog and still used it infrequently. It was five months since I quit using Humalog, but its effects keep rearing its head periodically, and I used the NovoLog to correct it. The effect I'm talking about is while exercising, my glucose does not want to fall as it should. I work out for an hour with weights, and sometimes I fail to perspire for a half hour and my glucose will not coming down. Once I begin to perspire, then I feel my glucose begin to fall. The effects of the NovoLog are now not as pronounced as they were when I first started taking it. This may be because I'm not taking as much as I was at first, and back then I also briefly took the Levemir insulin in the evening, which also hinders the liver from releasing glucose.

The papers you get with the Humalog give no information of importance and in fact seem to be a bit vague. They mention how insulin promotes anabolism, inhibits protein catabolism, and inhibits gluconeogenesis, but it implies at the beginning of the paragraph that all insulin have the same activities and the only difference with Humalog is that its effect is more rapid. However, from my years of using it, I feel it has the opposite effect that NovoLog has. NovoLog hinders the release of glucose by the liver, and Humalog promotes the release of glucose by the liver. What is most irritating about this is that according to doctors, there is no difference between the insulin; they both act the same way: quick acting, no difference—even though the papers with NovoLog and Levemir clearly state a difference. It may not be stated as a difference, but it is clearly a difference.

I don't know whether any studies have been done on any of these insulin or if there will be any in the future. I, right now, am sticking with the human insulin N and R. N insulin or NPH is just regular insulin with an isophane suspension to slow down its absorption or action of the insulin, but once the insulin is in action in the body, it is still the same regular insulin that is meant for the human body. Humalog, NovoLog, Apidra, Levemir, and Lantus are all what I refer to as engineered insulin, which are foreign to the body, and over time there is the potential for detrimental effects such as what I experienced and am still having a problem making it go away.

Since I stopped taking the Humalog insulin, all the problems with my diabetes have subsided. Morning syndrome only requires five to six units in the evening, and I also am not experiencing problems with my glucose controlled higher than what it should be. Apidra insulin is produced by Sanofi Aventis. I have never used it, but I believe it is similar to NovoLog in that it also hinders the liver from releasing glucose. Sanofi also makes the Lantus insulin that I used for a couple of years and was quite comfortable with. I considered it better than the Levemir and am not aware of any adverse effects on my liver. The only reason I quit using it was because my HMO insurance company was getting kickbacks from Novo Nordisk, so they stopped honoring any of the other insulin. So by eliminating all the engineered insulin, no one has any more control over me, not even the doctors who try to hold prescriptions over your head.

At one time, I didn't need any insulin in the evening—once in a while some regular at dinner but no long-duration insulin. I had hoped when I quit using Humalog insulin my diabetes would improve to the way it was before I started taking it. The progression of the insulin is so slow you never realize what is happening. I just felt it was a normal progression caused by aging.

Conclusion

As previously stated, I've been a diabetic for sixty years and am still quite healthy in spite of the medical profession. During my years with diabetes, I have seen numerous doctors, probably numbering twenty or more. Out of them, only one did me any good with my diabetes. That doctor was J. Deaver Alexander, and all the rest were nothing but useless, not only with my diabetes but with other problems I went to see them about.

I have had numerous problems as a diabetic, and they all went unresolved by the medical profession. I had to solve my own problems. Now first, my diabetes may have been caused by the medical world itself. My wife works with a person who, some time ago, told my wife this story about his younger brother. His younger brother was hit by a car in Philadelphia and was taken to a hospital. While in the hospital, the boy got, I believe, a staph infection. The doctors wanted to use penicillin to fight the infection but warned the boy's family that it might leave him with diabetes. They cured him of the infection, and indeed he became diabetic. I periodically tried to find information on diabetes being caused by penicillin since I was put on it while recovering from rheumatic fever.

I kept running into dead ends on the internet with the subject of penicillin causing diabetes, searching to no avail. Finally I searched with Bing and entered "diabetes caused by penicillin" and came across a website: AboutDiabetesInformation.com. The particular article I looked at was "Causes of Diabetes: Irregular and Unhealthy Eating Habits."

The article went on to say that many renowned researchers hold the belief that a deficiency of vitamin B6 may be a cause of diabetes. A lack of vitamin B causes the transformation of tryptophan (an amino acid present in our diet) into xanthurenic acid, which harms the beta cells of the pancreas to cause diabetes. It goes on to say that consumption of food containing excessive animal proteins, saturated fats, and calories also stimulates the production of xanthurenic acid in the body and that a similar effect is produced by the penicillin group of drugs. So at last I had some information that said quite possibly the medical profession and its treatment of rheumatic fever caused my diabetes. Even if I did have a strep infection, why assume I will get another one and try to prevent it with penicillin? It seems the medical profession tries to find whatever excuse it can to feed drugs to us without any regard for detrimental effects.

My next irritation with the medical profession came after Dr. Alexander's retirement. I was having a big problem with insulin shock at night. I sometimes didn't know where my glucose was before bedtime. Blood glucose monitoring for patients had just been developed. If it had been developed a few years previously, Dr. Alexander would have immediately introduced me to it, but I had to go through three doctors before getting any information about it. The reason for this was because that great organization (ha-ha), the AMA, wouldn't endorse the use of it until 1990, and once they did, they fed us bullshit. They said they had to ensure the lab accuracy of it. Ten years to analyze a product for reliability and accuracy? What a joke. When I was having problems with insulin shock at night, a poor estimate would have been better than nothing. But what do you expect from the AMA? My opinion, and a very correct opinion, is that the AMA finally had no choice but to endorse blood glucose monitoring for the patients because the cat was already out of the bag, and there was no stopping it. There were other doctors who did see the importance of blood glucose monitoring and recommended it to their patients in spite of the AMA. Also, I feel the AMA dragged their feet because they were afraid that the doctors who subscribed to them would lose control of patients with blood glucose monitoring in their hands, but it took their small minds ten years to understand that was not happening.

As far as lab accuracy goes, let's take a look at it. The lab that I am required to use by my insurance is Quest Diagnostics. For glucose, they have a range of sixty-five to ninety-nine, and American Medical Laboratories in Fairfax, Virginia, has a range of seventy to one hundred eighteen. I have results from other labs that fall in between these ranges. These two labs had the furthest spread in their ranges for the same test. Glucose is always measured for MG/DL, milligrams per deciliter. I've asked medical professionals before about this, and the answer I always got was they use a different test method. If that is true, then so much for lab accuracy. Of course, the more likely reason is that the medical profession can't decide on what the actual range of the test should be.

Previously in my history, I mentioned a problem with low triglycerides. At a local hospital's medical lab, they gave a range of forty to one hundred sixty. Quest labs designate their range as less than a hundred and fifty, and the range of another local hospital lab was twenty to a hundred and seventy. The labs all tested the same thing, MG/DL, and it bothers me that there can be such a wide variation of ranges in this test at various labs, especially the one lab that says it doesn't matter if there are any triglycerides in your body at all, which is what one doctor did say to me. In fact, his exact words were "The lower, the better." My own research at the library contradicted what he said, which I addressed in my history.

The next subject irritates me most of all, and most of this anger is directed at the FDA. It is about the MSG that the FDA allows the food industry to put in our food. It may not be life-threatening, but it causes so many bad reactions in people that it should be banned from use. It caused me two different stays in two different hospitals, with neither of them able to figure out what was wrong with me, and when my wife and I finally figured out what my problem was, my doctor at the time totally lied to me, trying to keep me stupid and blind to the real problem, which was MSG.

Back in 2011, there was a problem with food dyes that the food industry puts in our food to make it more appealing, especially to children. Some of the dyes have had a detrimental effect on children. Besides the psychological problems it induces, there is also a consumption problem it induces by being so much more appealing for consumption. We have a problem in this country with the overconsumption of junk food, and most of these foods with the coloring dyes administered are junk with little nutritional benefit. The only benefit of the coloring dyes is to make the food more appealing to the public so they can sell more and make everyone fatter. But our esteemed FDA's solution to the problem is warning labels, not an outright ban of the substances. Both MSG and food coloring have no benefit to anyone but the food industry. One does nothing but make food taste better without having to use legitimate spices, and the other makes their junk more appealing to eat, both at the detriment of us, the American public. But what does the FDA care? They don't work for us; they work for the food and pharmaceutical industries. They work for them and protect them. Since they don't work to protect us from them, why should the American taxpayer be required to pay their salaries? Let the food and pharmaceutical industries pay their salaries. When they screw up, the lawyers are what make them accountable, not the FDA. The FDA spends more time covering their butts and very little time protecting the public from bad drugs and questionable food additives. Let me back up a bit. From what I have learned in the past few years, the food industry and pharmaceutical companies do pay much of the FDA's salaries because the FDA charges fees for much of what they do for companies. I believe you can begin to see why FDA is so corrupt.

Let me summarize the medical problems I've had to resolve myself: Insulin shock in the middle of the night, of which I no longer have any since introducing myself to blood glucose monitoring. My problems with MSG with absolutely no help from the medical profession. In fact, my doctor insisted on being a detriment to me in resolving it. I was bitten by a tick that gave me Rocky Mountain spotted fever, which was resolved by a doctor who insisted mistakenly that I had Lyme disease. Fortunately for me, both diseases are treated with the same antibiotic, and it wasn't a severe case. I had problems with morning syndrome and had to resolve that myself. I broke my femur and the doctor wanted me on Coumadin and lied to me when I refused. The drug was totally unnecessary. After all, I did not take it, and I'm still here. Coumadin may be necessary for a rare few, but not for everyone. I'm sure there are other blood tests that could determine for whom it is necessary, but hell, that's money out of the pharmaceutical industry's pocket, and we can't have that. Right now I have a doctor who thinks all fast-action insulin are the same, and Levemir and Lantus are the same—no difference. It is important to understand the differences, but the doctors don't. Anyway, since the retirement of Dr. Alexander at the end of the seventies, I have been completely on my own without any assistance from the medical profession—not by my own choosing but because they gave me no choice but to turn my back on them. Why reward incompetence by following their orders and giving them money?

So far I have only addressed insulin-dependent diabetics. I know little about controlling diabetes on oral drugs and feel that very few people should be on the drugs. They impose great risk to everyone taking them. This opinion comes from the writings of other doctors and my own stepson's experience with the oral drugs. He was on Glucotrol and had high blood pressure problems and was extremely thin and couldn't put on any weight. His doctor kept upping his amount, but it did not benefit him much with the increases. He finally approached me as to what he should do. I told him to dump the idiot he was presently going to and find another doctor. I gave him the name of a doctor that I went to and liked but quit seeing because of a smug receptionist that she had working for her. Also, I told him to get off the oral drugs, that they are no good. He went and saw the doctor I recommended and told her he wanted to be on insulin. She agreed with him and put him on insulin. His blood pressure went back to 120 over 80, and his weight went back to normal. I don't know how long it took for everything to return to normal, but he says that even if he could, he would never take the oral medicines again. A few other points should be made about oral diabetic drugs. They all affect your heart to a degree. Watch your television. Seven or eight years ago there were notices on TV concerning Avandia being taken off the market. Avandia had, I believe, new controls and restrictions on the use of it. I don't believe it was completely removed from use, although in my opinion it should have been. There is a law firm that had advertisements asking people to call them if they have been on Avandia and suffered consequences. I believe there was another one previous to Avandia that was removed from use for causing too much harm to diabetics. Also, I have had a conversation with a salesperson for Sanofi Aventis who told me that they're instructed to encourage doctors to try to disengage patients from the oral drugs as soon as possible. Now of course they want them on their Lantus insulin for more customers and, of course, profit, but maybe they have genuine concerns for diabetics. After all, they, more than anyone, are likely to realize the dangers of the oral drugs and would like to promote people getting off them. Heart problems occur at a higher rate in diabetics than normal people, and I believe it is significantly higher. I haven't heard any statistics on it, but I would certainly like to see a statistic on the difference between oral control and insulin control concerning heart disease.

Since I'm on heart disease, next I would like to address statin drugs. My cholesterol is and most always been around 180—sometimes lower and sometimes a little over 200. This was probably driven by the AMA, but the attitude in the medical profession is that diabetics need to have their cholesterol below 150. I consider this complete garbage and have irritated a few doctors by telling them to shove their statin drugs, that my cholesterol is fine right where it is. There are plenty in the medical profession that say lowering your cholesterol is not going to have any effect on decreasing heart problems, and then there is the other side of the argument that says lower cholesterol is going to save your life. That side of the argument is presented by—who else? The statin drug industry and doctors who like to prescribe drugs. Statin drugs are loaded with many side effects such as memory loss, muscle discomfort, and others. The memory loss isn't mentioned much as a side effect of the statin drugs, which makes me wonder why. Maybe memory loss opens up another drug for the medical profession to administer. It is also my opinion that statin drugs are not what cause muscle discomforts but the lower cholesterol itself. This opinion comes from my own cholesterol-lowering experience.

About ten years ago I was experiencing discomfort in a few of my toes on my left foot. I didn't consult a doctor; I just felt it might be gout. So I read some articles about gout, and one article I read told about an old-time doctor who treated his patients with gout with an herb called stinging nettles with good success. So I decided to try it. After taking it for a couple of months, the discomfort in my toes disappeared, and I had an added benefit: it lowered my cholesterol to about 150. During my time of taking stinging nettles, which was for a couple of years, I experienced muscle discomfort, mostly in my arms and especially at the bottom of my spinal column. I mentioned this to my doctor, and his first response was x-rays, which I didn't bother with. A year later, at my next appointment, I had decided to quit taking the stinging nettles a month before the appointment. I did this so that my cholesterol would rise and cause some conflict with the doctor because he liked my cholesterol that low and just assumed it was due to eating habits. After I stopped taking stinging nettles, all the muscle discomfort I was experiencing went away after a couple of weeks. Of course, after tests prescribed by the doctor, it showed my cholesterol was back up to 190. This went totally unnoticed and unmentioned by the doctor. So much for trying to cause a conflict. The discomfort in my toes never returned, and I no longer take stinging nettles.

To conclude, if your cholesterol is below 200, I would not worry about pushing it lower, and certainly not with statin drugs.

What really appalls me about the medical profession in this country and the pharmaceutical business especially is how quick they are to develop a drug for every dumb ailment. The latest one is for gout. I don't remember what the drug is called and could care less, but it comes with cautions and side effects. If you have gout, take stinging nettles. No more gout and no side effects. You'll find it at your local health food store. Another treatment for gout that has developed over the past five years or more is tart cherry juice.

With the next six pages, I hope to do whatever I can to dispel a myth that too many people embrace in this country. It's a myth that causes me much irritation, and I hear it from politicians, people in general, and talk show hosts. This absurd myth is that we have the greatest healthcare system in the world. What irritates me the most about this pathetic belief is that as long as too many people, especially our politicians, believe this, nothing will improve, and after reading my history as a diabetic, I hope you feel there is a need and plenty of room for improvement. Study the next six pages, please, and think about the problems we have with our present system.

Total Health Expenditures as % of GDP, 2000 and 2008

The following table is derived from the data in the World Health Organization Statistical Information System. The 2011 report is available at http://www.who.int/whosis/. These statistics are from a previous book I have written, and although about ten years old, they will have changed insignificantly.

Total Health expenditure as % of GDP

Rank Country 2000-2008

1) United States of America 13.4 15.2
2) Marshall Islands 20.3 14.0
3) Nauru 11.3 14.0
4) Timor-Leste 8.8 13.9
5) Maldives 8.7 13.7
6) Niue 8.0 13.5
7) Micronesia (Fed. States of) 8.2 13.3
8) Kiribati 8.0 12.5
9) Cuba 6.7 12.0
10) France 10.1 11.2
11) Belgium 9.0 11.1
12) Palau 10.6 10.8
13) Switzerland 10.2 10.7
14) Portugal 8.8 10.6
15) Austria 9.9 10.5
16) Germany 10.3 10.5
17) Bosnia & Herzegovina 7.1 10.3
18) Greece 7.9 10.1

19) Denmark 8.3 9.9
20) Netherlands 8.0 9.9
21) Canada 8.8 9.8
22) New Zealand 7.7 9.7
23) Tuvalu 12.4 9.7
24) Sweden 8.2 9.4
25) Jordan 9.7 9.4
26) Iceland 9.8 9.2
27) Malawi 6.0 9.1
28) Spain 7.2 9.0
29) Finland 7.2 8.8
30) Georgia 7.0 8.7
31) Ireland 6.1 8.7
32) Italy 8.1 8.7
33) São Tomé & Principe 11.1 8.7
34) United Kingdom 7.0 8.7
35) Australia 8.0 8.5
36) Lebanon 10.7 8.5
37) Japan 7.7 8.3

Healthy Life Expectancy

The following table is derived from data in the world Health Organization Statistical Information System. These are estimates for people born in 2009.

Rank Country Total Male Female Population

1) Japan 83 80 86
2) San Marino 83 82 85
3) Andorra 82 79 85
4) Australia 82 80 84
5) Iceland 82 80 83
6) Israel 82 80 83
7) Italy 82 79 84

8) Monaco 82 78 85
9) Singapore 82 79 84
10) Spain 82 78 85
11) Switzerland 82 80 84
12) Canada 81 79 83
13) Cyprus 81 78 83
14) France 81 78 85
15) Luxembourg 81 78 83
16) Netherlands 81 78 83
17) New Zealand 81 79 83
18) Norway 81 79 83
19) Sweden 81 79 83
20) Austria 80 78 83
21) Belgium 80 77 83
22) Finland 80 77 83
23) Germany 80 78 83
24) Greece 80 78 83
25) Ireland 80 77 82
26) Malta 80 78 82
27) South Korea 80 77 83
28) United Kingdom 80 78 82
29) Chile 79 76 82
30) Costa Rica 79 77 81
31) Denmark 79 77 81
32) Portugal 79 76 82
33) Slovenia 79 76 82
34) United States 79 76 81
35) Cuba 78 76 80
36) Czech Republic 77 74 80
37) Panama 77 74 79
38) Marshall Islands 59 58 60

I listed the Marshall Islands without a rank because there are many countries with a life expectancy between seventy-seven and fifty-nine, but it intrigues me that Marshall Islands is second to the United States in health expenditures yet ranks so low in life expectancy.

Under 5 Mortality Rate

Again this table is derived from WHO statistics and is from 2009 levels from their 2011 report available at http://www.who.int/whosis/.

Rank Country under 5 Mortality Rate / Stillborn

1,000 live births births / 1,000

1) Luxembourg 2 3
2) San Marino 2 3
3) Finland 3 2
4) Iceland 3 2
5) Singapore 3 2
6) Cyprus 3 3
7) Japan 3 3
8) Slovenia 3 3
9) Sweden 3 3
10) Denmark 4 2
11) Germany 4 2
12) Norway 4 2
13) Andorra 4 3
14) Czech Republic 4 3
15) Greece 4 3
16) Ireland 4 3
17) Italy 4 3
18) Monaco 4 3
19) Portugal 4 3
20) Spain 4 3
21) Switzerland 4 3
22) Estonia 4 4
23) France 4 4
24) Australia 5 3
25) Belgium 5 3
26) Israel 5 3
27) Netherlands 5 3

28) South Korea 5 3
29) Austria 5 4
30) United Kingdom 5 4
31) Canada 6 3
32) Croatia 6 3
33) Poland 6 3
34) Hungary 6 4
35) Lithuania 6 4
36) Cuba 6 8
37) Malta 7 3
38) Slovakia 7 4
39) United Arab Emirates 7 4
40) Serbia 7 5
41) Montenegro 8 3
42) United States 8 3
43) Latvia 8 4
44) Chile 8 9

Maternal Mortality Ratio

This table is derived from WHO statistics and is from 2008 levels from their 2011 report.

Rank Country Maternal Mortality ratio/100,000

1) Greece 2
2) Ireland 3
3) Austria 5
4) Belgium 5
5) Denmark 5
6) Iceland 5
7) Italy 5
8) Sweden 5
9) Japan 6
10) Slovakia 6
11) Spain 6

12) Germany 7
13) Israel 7
14) Norway 7
15) Portugal 7
16) Australia 8
17) Czech Republic 8
18) Finland 8
19) France 8
20) Malta 8
21) Qatar 8
22) Serbia 8
23) Kuwait 9
24) Netherlands 9
25) Singapore 9
26) Cyprus 10
27) Switzerland 10
28) United Arab Emirates 10
29) Estonia 12
30) Canada 12
31) United Kingdom 12
32) Bulgaria 13
33) Hungary 13
34) Lithuania 13
35) Croatia 14
36) New Zealand 14
37) Belarus 15
38) Montenegro 15
39) Luxembourg 17
40) Slovenia 18
41) South Korea 18
42) Bahrain 19
43) Latvia 20
44) Oman 20
45) Turkey 23
46) Saudi Arabia 24
47) United States 24

48) Chile 26
49) Lebanon 26
50) China 39
51) Russia 38

The previous tables are estimates done by the World Health Organization. For more complete listings and a better understanding of these statistics, go to http://www.who.int/whosis/.

Mortality Amenable to Healthcare or Preventable Deaths

This table is derived from a study supported by the Commonwealth Fund, which included nineteen countries and was done over two study periods in 1997–98 and 2002–03. It compared preventable deaths.

% Deaths per 100,000 Population

Rank Country 1997–98 2002–03

1) France 76 65
2) Japan 81 71
3) Australia 88 71
4) Spain 84 74
5) Italy 89 74
6) Canada 89 77
7) Norway 99 80
8) Netherlands 97 82
9) Sweden 88 82
10) Greece 97 84
11) Austria 109 84
12) Germany 106 90
13) Finland 116 93
14) New Zealand 115 96
15) Denmark 113 101
16) United Kingdom 130 103
17) Ireland 134 103

18) Portugal   128   104
19) United States   115   110

The rate of amenable mortality is considered a valuable indicator of healthcare performance. Data for this study comes from the World Health Organization on deaths from conditions considered amenable to healthcare, such as treatable diseases. In this study, the United States rated last among the nineteen nations selected for the study. Not only that, the United States showed the least improvement between the two periods, ranking sixteenth in the first period and last in the second period. This study was done by two American doctors.

World's Health Systems Rankings

This table is derived from the WHO World Health Report from 2000. The rankings are for 1997 and were based on eight different categories. No more up-to-date rankings from WHO were available. They stopped doing these rankings due to their complexity.

Rank Country

1) France
2) Japan
3) San Marino
4) Andorra
5) Malta
6) Singapore
7) Spain
8) Oman
9) Austria
10) Italy
11) Norway
12) Portugal
13) Monaco
14) Greece
15) Iceland

16) Luxembourg
17) Netherlands
18) United Kingdom
19) Ireland
20) Switzerland
21) Belgium
22) Colombia
23) Sweden
24) Cyprus
25) Germany
26) Saudi Arabia
27) United Arab Emirates
28) Israel
29) Morocco
30) Canada
31) Finland
32) Australia
33) Chile
34) Denmark
35) Dominica
36) Costa Rica
37) United States
38) Slovenia
39) Cuba
40) Brunei Darussalam
41) New Zealand
42) Bahrain
43) Croatia
44) Qatar
45) Kuwait
46) Russia
47) China

Our country, the United States, leads the world in healthcare expenditures, but we don't even rank in the top ten in any of the categories that measure how good our health-care system is. I consider that appalling, and what's even more appalling is how politicians and talk show hosts feed us crap about how our system is the best in the world. I wonder what they base their empty rhetoric on, because empty is what it indeed is. They also like to state that all the other people of the world come to the United States for complicated or life-threatening procedures. Some indeed do, but rest assured, there are other countries that people go to for help with severe medical conditions. After all, the first heart transplant was not performed in the United States but in the Union of South Africa, and the first full facial transplant wasn't performed here either but in Spain. These two countries were pioneers in very complicated procedures. To think we are the only ones capable of saving the lives of other people throughout the world who are stricken with complicated medical problems is ludicrous.

Japan ranks thirty-sixth in health-care expenditures and number one in life expectancy, number two in preventable deaths, and is tied for number three in infant mortality rate. They're in the top ten in every category. If I were to say who has the best health-care system in the world, I would have to say it is Japan. Take a good look at the statistics; wouldn't you agree? Maybe what we need to do in this country is take our arrogance about how we have the best health-care system and shove it! Next, we should take a look at Japan's health-care system and other countries that do better than we do and see if we can't learn something from them. Of course, in order to learn something, we first have to get rid of the arrogance, and our medical profession has plenty of it. They teach arrogance to the medical students in college. When you have a chance, watch the movie *Patch Adams*, starring Robin Williams. It will leave you with an understanding of what I just stated about arrogance being taught by medical colleges.

My next criticism is of you, the public. Ten or twelve years ago, Regis Philbin, the one who had the television show in the morning, went through, I believe, bypass surgery on his heart.

When returning to his show after his recovery, he received emails, I guess, from fans, and he went over some of them. I rarely watch Regis, but I did that morning and was irritated by one letter that was sent to him. The person told Regis to listen to and obey everything the doctors told him. This advice from people has always been very irritating to me. What it says is submit to the doctors and let them have their way with you. If you paid attention to my history as a diabetic, you should be in some agreement with me when I say if I followed that advice, I doubt that I would be writing this book today. As I've stated before, doctors should be nothing more than advisors, and not in control of you. You have to take control of your life and be in charge. Listen to the advice of doctors, but accept it with an open mind and the realization that after you think about it and do some research, you might reject it. Sometimes, after decisions you make, you have to kick yourself in the ass, but when the bad decision has been made by your doctor, how do you go about kicking him in the ass? Telling him he was wrong won't accomplish much. They tend to reject any of your opinions. It's what they are taught in medical school. Any of your opinions on your medical well-being are irrelevant and should be discarded. How do you feel and what aches or pains you? Other than that, they don't want to hear anything from you, and they also don't want you to get any information that might allow you to develop an opinion of your own. Not all doctors are like this, but many are, and when you have one of these doctors, find another. I would also like to add that my opinion about how many good doctors there are is somewhere between 5 and 10 percent. This will be highly disputed, but the following paragraphs have some more statistics on the greatness of our medical system and the great strides in improving it and how great our doctors are.

In 1999, deaths caused by hospital medical errors were 98,000. The latest statistic that I read on deaths caused by hospitals has climbed to 195,000. Now let's look at the doctors. Doctors are the third-leading cause of death in the United States. About 250,000 deaths per year are caused by doctor-related medical errors. In July of 2000, a report appeared in the *Journal of the American Medical Association* (July 26; vol. 284 no. 4, pp. 483–485). This report is ten years old but discusses the problems doctors cause. Now I know I have previously denounced the AMA, but their journal is composed of articles written by medical professionals who aren't run-of-the-mill doctors. I also imagine that there is some overlap in hospital-caused deaths and doctor-related deaths, because I don't know the specifics on how hospital-related-death data is compiled. I would hope deaths caused by doctor errors are not considered the fault of the hospital.

As you can see, there has been no improvement in hospital care in the past ten years. In fact, our care is in decline. Hospital staff infection occurrences have not declined, and the severity of the infections has increased. Hospital administrators are very lax in implementing any safeguards to ensure the safety and well-being of patients, according to a few articles I have read on the subject. One of the articles gave a reason that I don't fully recall. One article described procedures that needed to be implemented and didn't want to step on any toes in its explanation of why they weren't implemented. My explanation of why they were not implemented is much simpler than theirs: laziness justified by arrogance and, of course, stupidity. One other point the article made was of the cost savings if the procedures were implemented. They weren't specific about who would enjoy the cost savings—whether it would be the hospital or the patients. I believe it would be both, most certainly the patients. One simple procedure is cleanliness. How often do the nurses and the doctors wash their hands? As a patient, you should be aware of this by simply asking the nurses and your doctor.

Deaths caused by hospital mistakes have increased by 60 percent in just the past two years. Our medical system is in shambles and certainly not getting better. First and foremost, what prevents any improvement in the system is the arrogance of most of the ones that make up the medical profession, and like I previously said, it is taught to them by small-minded people in medical college. The greatest minds are not the ones who teach. That arrogance is also perpetuated by the constant garbage from news people, advertisements, and people in general. Listen to your doctor and obey your doctor's orders. In some cases, a patient is so stupid that he does, indeed, need to follow that advice, but it is not good advice for all. If you are a thinking person, what "obey your doctor's orders" is supposed to mean to you is "quit thinking and do as your doctor says, because he knows best and you know nothing," but the two previous paragraphs dispute that, wouldn't you agree?

"Listen to your doctor, he knows best, obey your doctor, we've got the best medical system in the world." All this is garbage fed to us to keep us in line, and this bullshit is constantly fed to us even by ourselves, but the statistics, which are very factual, show a very different picture. The reason why they paint this rosy picture is because the stupider they keep us, the easier it is to keep fleecing us. The fleecing is by the entire mainstream medical profession: doctors, hospitals, and most of all, the pharmaceutical industry.

The United States and New Zealand are the only countries that allow advertisements on television by the pharmaceutical industry. Allowing them to advertise is not a good idea except for the drug companies. When something ails you, your first action should be to visit your doctor and have him diagnose your problem and then decide the best line of treatment, and in some cases that is still the way it is done. In many cases, though, you see an advertisement on TV and go to your doctor and say I need a prescription for this drug. The doctor may disagree but has a problem with giving you much of an argument on it because he has to risk you going somewhere else in order to get the drug. I am all for second-guessing doctors, but not when it is to get drugs. Second-guess them when it comes to refusing them, not so you can get them. A natural drug-free solution should be your priority. After all, do any of you pay attention to the drug advertisements? At the end of all of them is a brief statement, usually not complete, about side effects. The final statement almost always says your kidneys and liver will have to be checked to make sure there are no problems with either. If those organs have to be healthy before starting use, what do you think is likely to happen after prolonged use? Can you imagine how much money they're going to harvest from you if they do destroy your kidneys or liver or both? And believe me, they could care less. To them it's the money that is important.

Everyone wants to think their doctor cares about them, and many actually think they do and their doctor will tell them how concerned they are about them, but face facts. You're not a personal friend or family, just a person to get money to come from your pocket into theirs. After all, do you ever have any kind of personal conversation with any of them? When they prescribe drugs to you, it's the easiest way for them to do their job. It takes little thought, and you have to keep coming back for monitoring of the drug and/or renewals. Doctors are basically trained drug pushers and little else. In fact, an article that appeared in the newspaper a few years back told of a medical study done on doctors. It concerned heart monitoring and said many doctors are incapable of detecting defects when they listen to your heart. I don't remember the percentage, but it was significant and, to me, a bit alarming. The big heart problems were easily detected by most doctors, but it stated that most missed the more subtle warning signs.

Most doctors are quick to prescribe drugs and will only give natural treatment suggestions when you refuse their drug treatments and will have disdain for you afterward. But all drugs have side effects, and many have serious side effects. Of course, they always have another drug to relieve the side effect. Drugs should only be used as a last resort, but many doctors use them as the first resort. Hippocrates said that a doctor first should do no harm, and I believe it is in the Hippocratic Oath that doctors supposedly take. I don't even know whether they take that oath or ever did, but if they do take the oath, it's only a formality, without substance. Of course, this is my opinion. If the oath still means anything, then with so many side effects, why would a doctor's first response to any problem you have be to prescribe a drug when in many cases a nutritional approach would be more suitable? In most cases, the drugs only mask the symptoms, in many cases with consequences, where a nutritional approach eliminates the problem and without side effects. A perfect example is osteoarthritis, from which I used to suffer. I now take OsteoEZ, a nutritional supplement, and arthritis is no longer a problem for me. I may have a little insignificant stiffness every once in a while, but that is all. All the time that I was taking formulas of glucosamine sulfate, chondroitin, and MSM, which make up most of the store shelf supplements for arthritis seven or eight years ago, it bothered me by constant articles in the newspapers about studies done by medical schools that would state how ineffective the three components were. Finally an article came out in the newspaper about a study done by the federal government that stated glucosamine sulfate, chondroitin, and MSM were effective with 90 percent of the people who take them. After that, I hadn't seen any more articles on bogus medical school studies, sponsored by either the drug companies themselves or the AMA or both in conjunction with each other. Osteo Bi-Flex and other products on the market are not overnight fixes. You didn't wake up one morning with joint problems; it took a long time to wear out your joints so don't expect to rebuild them in a short period of time. The problem will be repaired though, and it is a much better solution than taking anything mainstream medicine has to offer, which is basically painkillers to mask the problem instead of getting rid of the problem.

What is most irritating about what I have just described is the great lengths that mainstream medicine (the AMA and their buddies, the drug companies) will go through to convince us that nutritional supplements are a waste of money. Two organizations I consider a waste of money, which are sidekicks of the drug companies and the AMA, are the American Diabetes Association (ADA) and the American Cancer Society (ACS). They both may make you feel good by giving money to them, but it is money flushed down the drain.

First, let's take a look at the ADA. When I first became a diabetic, my parents subscribed to a magazine of theirs called *Forecast*. In this magazine, they constantly would say how a cure for diabetes was right around the corner. That was sixty years ago, and I don't see any end to that corner yet. If you do need to give to something, then give to the Juvenile Diabetes Foundation and not the ADA. In the 1980s, when I first discovered the benefits of amino acids with my diabetes—and I mean the lowering of my insulin requirements from 120 units a day down to thirty units a day—there were problems I encountered, and all I got from any of the doctors was ignorance and stupidity. Ignorance is the lack of knowledge, and stupidity is the lack of a brain, and that was what I was confronted with, so I felt I would give the ADA a call and see if there was the presence of any intelligence there. I wanted to know from them if there was any research being done into the use of amino acids in the treatment of diabetes and tried to explain the benefits I got from them. All I received in response was "Your kidneys are already under stress from your diabetes.

Why would you take amino acids when it is going to stress them more?" I couldn't get anywhere in the conversation because they had no interest in anything I had to say. To them, I absolutely didn't know what I was talking about, and the conversation was abruptly ended.

It just further amazed me the fear that most of the medical world has of nutritional supplements. Before this happened, I was already aware of this fear from an interview that Bryant Gumbel had with an AMA spokesman on one of the morning news shows. This person from the AMA was talking about a legislation the AMA wanted to have passed outlawing all nutritional supplement stores, I guess banning all vitamins, herbs, or any nutritional supplements from being sold entirely. Mr. Gumbel cleverly asked what the problem was since they weren't allowed to advertise, and this person replied that other doctors write about the benefits from taking supplements, so they get advertising through the back door. This interview always intrigued me because this representative of the AMA was either the biggest moron in the world or was a plant to promote nutritional supplements. After all, that was what he actually did in my opinion. Presently 50 percent of the population takes some kind of nutritional supplement—hooray! I hope that percentage continues to grow, because in my mind, the benefits are astounding, and I can't understand why so many in the medical world are having such a problem coming to grips with it. Actually, I do. It's really very simple: there's much more money in peddling drugs than promoting nutritional health. There are doctors though that do promote nutritional supplements, and the number of them is increasing, but slowly.

With nutritional health, there is no money in it for the drug companies. The demise of our health-care system is generated directly by the pharmaceutical industry, and the FDA works for them and not for us. Seeing as they work for the drug companies and not us, their salaries should be paid by the drug companies and the food industry, not us. As far as controlling indiscretions by both industries, the lawyers and our courts have done more to control them than the FDA has. After all, why are there so many class action lawsuits advertised by the legal profession concerning products from the drug companies, and why have there been so many food recalls? When investigated, it seemed as if the FDA and USDA inspectors were visiting for a morning cup of coffee rather than doing their jobs as inspectors. Sometimes citations were issued but then ignored by both the ones receiving the citation and the FDA and the USDA themselves. The only way our health-care system can ever be improved is by stepping on both the drug industry and the food industry by stopping their abuses. In the food industry, this can be done by not allowing them their immense freedom to add whatever junk they wish to junk food to entice us, and especially our kids, to eat it. Sometimes additives are added to make us want to eat more of it. The FDA will do nothing to curtail this.

Now let me address my feelings toward the ACS and our immense cancer industry in general. One thing that infuriates me while watching television (something I don't do much of, but I do watch the news) is to see so many advertisements by hospitals concerning cancer. Cancer cures still remain at a dismal 5 percent at best, but listening to all these advertisements you'd think they're curing everyone. Well, they're not. Five percent is a dismal cure rate. They all make it sound like they have all these different treatment options when they don't. It's all the same old, same old, known by any forward-thinking doctor as slash, burn, poison, or otherwise known as operate, radiate, and chemo. All these have abhorrent cure rates and, in most cases, nonexistent cure rates and abhorrent side effects. As far as I am concerned, in most cases, people would be better off to accept death rather than go through the discomfort of chemotherapy because the sad truth of the treatment is that death is the end result anyway. All the hospitals like Cancer Treatment Centers of America and many other hospitals give these great advertisements that lead you to think that they are curing people of cancer when they're not. All these hospitals have nothing to offer but the same—operate, radiate, and chemo, otherwise known as slash, burn, poison. They all tell you about their diversity of treatments, but their diversity goes only as far as slash, burn, poison. There is nothing else that they have to offer. Their advertisements are nothing but a snow job. I've researched this by calling a few of the hospitals that have television advertisements to find out if they offer any alternative treatments, and they don't. I asked one person if they were allowed to give any information on alternative treatments other than operate, radiate, and poison, or would they get shut down by the FDA if they did give out alternative treatment information? She replied that she didn't think that they would go that far, but they sure do frown upon it.

The FDA has only one goal when it comes to cancer treatment, and that is to make sure the slash, burn, poison industry continues harvesting great amounts of money from the public. These people don't care whether this money is flushed down the drain without any benefit to us. I have watched family and other people that I knew go through conventional cancer treatment. All medicine did for them was prolong their lives with a great deal of discomfort and, in some cases, outright suffering. When you read in the newspapers about a new chemotherapy drug, what the article will state about its benefits is how much longer people will survive on the new drug. There is never any better cure percentage that they give, because they flat-out don't cure. The only benefit from the new chemo drug that they can talk about is the extended survival time. This is generally stated in terms of a few months that a person will now survive with their cancer. Never is a cure rate given because there is none. *Questioning Chemotherapy*, a book written by Dr. Ralph Moss, PhD, states that chemo is effective in only 2 to 4 percent of cancers, those being Hodgkin's disease, acute lymphocytic leukemia, testicular cancer, and choriocarcinoma.

The ACS always wants us contributing money to them to find a cure but sponsors no research in natural cures and has no information on alternative treatments. I have talked to one of their spokespersons over the phone. She told me that she would email me some information and also gave me a website to go to. I never received any email, and the website only offered different chemotherapy treatments available. Wouldn't you think a charity like the ACS would have information on alternative treatments and nutritional treatments with some kind of statistics compiled on it? No! All they are is an organization that it seems to me has nothing to give. On the website of the ACS, they state in their heading that they are the sponsor of birthdays. Bullshit!

If any of you reading this book have any concerns about cancer, arm yourself with knowledge. There are many good sources of information that I believe everyone should become familiar with and not wait until you are at the mercy of the medical profession. The only information or advice they will give and in fact are only allowed to give you is the conventional slash, burn, poison treatments. Protect yourself and read about cancer. Myself, I have read *Knockout* by Suzanne Somers, and off the internet I downloaded a book that anyone can download by entering into Bing or Google "Michael Cutler, MD." On his website is his book titled *A Doctor's Treasury of Once-Censored Cancer Cures*. Another website worth looking at is http://germancancerbreakthrough.com, from Andrew Scholberg. This website is an advertisement for his book with the same title, and by the way, he tells in his book how President Ronald Reagan secretly went to Germany in May of 1985 and was treated for cancer and cured. We all know when President Reagan died nineteen years later; it was not from cancer. All three of these books, as far as I'm concerned, are must-read. All three will enlighten you to how we are being ripped off by mainstream medicine under the protection of the FDA and the complicity of the American Cancer Society. Previously when I said the medical profession is only allowed to give you information on slash, burn, poison, that is because of the FDA. The FDA could care a damn about us. They only care about protecting the pharmaceutical industry, the radiation industry, and the hospitals. As long as they keep harvesting money from us and us having little to show for it, the FDA is content that they have been doing their job very well.

There are other good websites concerning cancer that you can research on your own. One other that I would like to mention is www.cancerfightingstrategies.com, and of course if you think mainstream medicine is the only way to go, they have plenty of websites also. Most of this research into websites was done by me around 2010 or 2011. They may not still exist.

Obamacare! This massive piece of legislation that Rep. Pelosi from California said we have to pass it so we can find out what's in it. It's two thousand pages of trash, and we still barely know what's in it. So far all it has accomplished is to force the insurance business to no longer deny people coverage and extend coverage of your children, to put it as briefly as possible. But with these benefits, everyone's insurance policies are going to cost more. After all, insurance companies are not working on the high profit margin that all the medical industry works on, so they can't just pull money out of their ass to pay for this extra coverage dictated by the federal government.

Meaningful legislation meant to improve our dismal medical system is an impossible thing to expect. You see, a bit of information I got from Michael Cutler's book is that in the last ten years, forty-two senators have invested money in the pharmaceutical industry. Do you really think that we will see any legislation that will curtail the profits of the drug companies? The drug companies do not need our medical system improved because if it is, it will cut into their profits; any improvement has to start with the drug companies. One recent bit of news that came out was that 80 percent of all the pain medicines in the world are consumed here in the United States. That is a pathetic statistic; as a proud citizen of this country, it makes me a bit ashamed, but honestly, do you think Big Pharma would like to see that statistic curtailed or that any of our esteemed senators would like to see it curtailed? I don't think so!

With almost half of the Senate with money invested in the drug business and our former Speaker of the House making such an idiotic remark about passing the health-care bill so we can find out what is in it and the next Speaker of the House John Boehner stating that we have the best medical system in the world, I don't see much of a chance of any improvements being made in it. In fact, although there are problems that do need to be addressed in our medical system, I don't have any faith in our political system to recognize them and correct them. The first and biggest problem, in my opinion, is that our medical system overemphasizes the use of drugs for every medical problem. Drugs rarely eliminate problems but only camouflage the problem, and if they do eliminate a problem, they frequently create other problems. If we don't overemphasize the use of drugs, then please tell me why 80 percent of all pain medicine throughout the world is consumed by the United States.

Drugs don't make us a healthier nation, but less healthy. Of course, this is what the entire medical system wants. If we were a healthier nation, we would need to see doctors less, and fewer prescriptions for drugs would be needed. I do, however, see some improvement among doctors who actually are looking more toward resolving problems through nutrition and nutritional supplements and some who are turning their backs on the AMA. But there are still far too many who are still practicing the archaic mainstream way and who continuously try to denigrate nutritional supplements.

I take an assortment of nutritional supplements; the only medicine I take is insulin, and none of the engineered insulin. I also managed to decrease my insulin dosages from 120 units per day down to thirty to forty units per day, and I have kept it that low for the past twenty years or more. I have also driven it down to twenty units per day but have not been able to keep it that low. I experiment with my diabetes and don't consult with doctors in doing so. I used to try to talk to doctors about what I do with nutritional supplements, but the only response I would ever get is that it won't do any harm, but it won't do any good either. This was always the depth of the conversation, so why should I take any time to converse with the medical profession? With any medical problem, you have to take control of your life and not turn your life over to the doctors. Believe me when I say that few of them know what's best for you. Consult with them, but you must stay in control and make the final decision of what you do yourself.

In closing my book, I would like to address something that occurred the beginning of 2010 that infuriated me. A young man whom I believe was in his early teens had been stricken with cancer but was refusing chemotherapy treatment with the consent of his parents. The young man refused chemo because of the discomfort it caused him, and also he and his parents didn't believe any benefit would come of it and had more faith in alternative treatment. The doctors and hospital took the parents to court under the disguise of bad parenting, and the court ruled in favor of the medical establishment. The young man had to submit to chemotherapy. The young man himself and his parents now had no control over his condition. The medical profession could have their way. In my opinion, this case should have never come to court, and no judge should have made a ruling in favor of mainstream medicine. In some cases, parents refuse medical treatment for their child and the courts need to step in, but this was not the case in this incident. This family wanted to pursue other treatments. Our court system, though, decided that the only ones entitled to their money were the chemo industry, an industry with an abysmal record of curing cancer.

You have to analyze this case and wonder just where the control of our own lives is going and the control of our lives that the medical profession demands to have. If you give any thought to this, I'm sure you will be as appalled as I am with it. Something else that occurred some time ago was a letter that was sent in to our local newspaper by a person from Frazer, Pennsylvania. It was from a person who was with a group of people who were working on a project concerning elevating the body's temperature as a means of fighting cancer. Their funding was stopped. I don't remember whether the ACS and the FDA were involved, but quite frankly, they would have to be. This equipment has been developed in Germany and is in use in Germany and also by a doctor in Tijuana, Mexico. They are curing people of cancer with this system and only need to administer 10 percent of the chemotherapy that is normally given to cancer patients. There is no hair loss and no suffering from the effects of massive amounts of chemo. Unfortunately, this system will never be seen in the United States because of the FDA. One thing that intrigues me is whether the man from Frazer packed up and went to Germany to develop his system for fighting cancer or whether Germany was already working on one of their own. One thing that has to be understood is that Germany allows alternative treatments, something that is not allowed in the United States. If he did go to Germany, wouldn't it have been better to keep those jobs and technology here in America? This treatment was perceived because a woman back in 1880s or 1890s was suffering with melanoma skin cancer, and during her treatment, she got the flu and ran a high fever. Once she was over the flu and her fever subsided, her doctor noticed her melanoma cancer was gone also. The doctor credited the fever in getting rid of the cancer. So way back in the end of the 1800s, we were aware of the effect of heat on cancer. This treatment has been developed but excluded from use in the United States. Where does the FDA get off preventing this system from being used in this country? Like I said, they work for the pharmaceutical industry and not us. Human life means nothing to the FDA. The only thing that matters to them is the profits of the pharmaceutical industry and, in this situation, the chemo business.

I hope with my conclusion that you have developed a better understanding of the medical profession. I don't mean to have you turn your back on them completely because I, by no means, have, but I don't see them and let them have their way with me. I am suggesting that you question everything and take nothing for granted with them.

www.ingramcontent.com/pod-product-compliance
Lightning Source LLC
LaVergne TN
LVHW091558060526
838200LV00036B/897